The
Timeless Guide
Secrets to a Long and Healthy Life

By
Dr. Sage Evergreen

The
Timeless Guide
Secrets to a Long and Healthy Life

Table of Contents

Introduction

We all want to live longer, healthier lives, don't we? The quest for longevity isn't just about adding years to your life; it's about adding life to your years. When your body and mind are in harmony, life becomes a series of joyful, fulfilling experiences rather than a struggle against time. In this book, we're embarking on a journey to explore how you can achieve that harmony and optimize both your health and your lifespan.

The concept of longevity might seem like a modern obsession, but the desire to extend human life has existed for centuries. Philosophers, scientists, and everyday people have pondered the secrets to a long, vibrant life. In contemporary times, scientific advancements have brought us closer than ever to understanding the mechanics behind aging and how to influence them. You're not just at the mercy of your genes; your environment, lifestyle choices, and mindset play crucial roles. Our goal here is to crack the code of longevity with actionable, evidence-based strategies.

Imagine waking up each day with boundless energy, a sharp mind, and a body that moves with ease. Picture yourself enjoying activities you love, surrounded by people who inspire you, all while feeling an inner sense of peace. Sounds pretty dreamy, right? Well, that can be your reality. This is not a pipe dream but a reachable goal. With the right information, you can make small but impactful changes to improve your quality of life significantly.

Your journey to a healthier, longer life won't require a radical overhaul of your current lifestyle, but it will demand intention and commitment. You don't have to do it alone, though. This book is here as your guiding star, offering you insights into the science of aging, nutrition, exercise, mental health, and much more.

We're going to dive deep into how you can enhance your lifespan through nutrition, focusing on the power of whole foods and the benefits of superfoods and fasting. You'll learn how specific dietary choices can stave off inflammation and oxidative stress, two major culprits in the aging process. Hinging on this nutritional foundation, we'll explore the best exercises for longevity, encompassing strength training, cardiovascular health, and flexibility. No, you don't need to become a gym rat, but a well-rounded fitness routine can make all the difference.

Equally important is your mental health. Chronic stress, poor sleep, and a lack of mindfulness can degrade your quality of life significantly. This book will provide practical tips for managing stress, improving sleep hygiene, and cultivating mindfulness, helping you build mental resilience and emotional stability. Your mental well-being is just as critical as your physical health in the quest for longevity. Remember, a peaceful mind contributes to a healthy body.

But let's not stop there. We'll delve into the power of social connections in Chapter 5. The benefits of having a strong support network and meaningful relationships cannot be overstated. Humans are inherently social beings, and loneliness can negatively impact both your mental and physical health. You'll learn how to build and maintain a supportive social network, enriching your life and those around you.

Next, we'll explore environmental factors and how they play into your overall health. Creating a healthy home environment and reducing your exposure to toxins can significantly improve your well-being. Often, the small things we overlook have the biggest impact.

Chapter 7 links ancient wisdom with modern science. You might find solace in traditional medicine practices or holistic approaches that align with contemporary findings. These intertwined modalities can offer a comprehensive path to wellness.

In the realm of personalized medicine, genetic testing and tailored health protocols promise a new era of individualized care. No two individuals are the same, and a one-size-fits-all approach to health and longevity simply won't cut it in today's world. You'll discover how personalized strategies can address your unique needs, maximizing your potential for a long and healthy life.

Preventative healthcare is our next focus, demonstrating the importance of regular check-ups and early detection strategies. Your future self will thank you for taking proactive steps today. Prevention is indeed better than cure.

What truly makes life worth living is having a sense of purpose and passion. In Chapter 10, you'll learn how finding meaning and pursuing what lights you up can contribute to a longer, more satisfying life. Passion fuels your spirit and invigorates your body, serving as a catalyst for longevity.

Real-life stories always serve as powerful testimonials. In Chapter 11, we'll share interviews with centenarians and lessons from the long-lived. These aren't just tales of luck but stories of intent and wise choices. Their experiences are beacons guiding you on your journey.

The last chapter offers actionable tips for everyday living. From morning routines to evening wind-downs and goal setting, you'll have practical advice to incorporate into your daily life. The small habits you adopt can lead to dramatic changes over time.

We are standing on the precipice of an exciting era where living longer and better is attainable for more people than ever before. This is your time to harness the wisdom and resources available to you. Ready to start?

Chapter 1:
The Science of Longevity

Imagine living a life where each day is filled with vitality and purpose, regardless of your age. The science of longevity isn't just a distant dream but a tangible reality that's unfolding through groundbreaking research and innovative health strategies. By understanding the complex mechanisms of aging and identifying key biomarkers, science reveals powerful insights that can significantly extend our healthy years. As we dive into the fascinating realm of longevity, brace yourself for a journey that blends the rigor of scientific inquiry with the practical wisdom of everyday life. We're talking about harnessing the power of your own biology, making informed decisions, and embracing holistic wellness practices that can lead to a longer, richer life. Let's uncover the secrets that can help us not just to add years to our lives, but life to our years.

Understanding Aging

Aging—it's something we all experience but seldom understand, really. It's a complex process influenced by a combination of genetic, biological, and environmental factors. As we start peeling back the layers, the goal here isn't just to slow growing old; it's about mastering the art of growing older in a way that optimizes health and longevity. So, how do we make sense of this multifaceted phenomenon that touches every corner of our lives?

Aging isn't merely about turning the pages of the calendar. It involves intricate biochemical processes that affect our cells, tissues, and organs. At its core, aging is the result of accumulating cellular damage over time. But don't let that scare you—understanding these processes can empower you to make choices that defy the typical aging narrative. Essentially, think of aging as a finely tuned orchestra, where each section needs to be in sync for the symphony of life to play beautifully.

One of the most fascinating aspects of aging is how it's influenced by both our genes and our environment. You've probably heard people say, "Oh, it's in my genes," when referring to their health or longevity. There is truth to that, but it isn't the whole story. Your genetic makeup indeed sets the stage, yet how the performance unfolds depends significantly on environmental factors like diet, exercise, stress levels, and even social connections.

At the cellular level, aging is marked by several key processes. First, there's the shortening of telomeres, the protective caps at the ends of your chromosomes. Each time a cell divides, these telomeres get a bit shorter, until they can no longer protect the chromosomes, leading to cellular aging and death. While this sounds grim, recent research shows that lifestyle choices can impact the rate of telomere shortening.

Additionally, oxidative stress plays a crucial role in aging. It's caused by free radicals—unstable molecules produced during normal cellular activities. Without adequate antioxidant defenses, these free radicals can damage DNA, proteins, and cells, accelerating the aging process. But guess what? Antioxidants found in whole foods can help neutralize these free radicals, offering a line of defense against oxidative stress.

Let's not overlook one more significant factor: inflammation. Chronic low-level inflammation, often dubbed "inflammaging," is a silent driver of aging and many age-related diseases. This inflammation can be triggered by various factors like poor diet, lack of exercise, and even emotional stress. Reducing inflammation through dietary choices, regular physical activity, and stress management is pivotal for healthy aging.

The role of mitochondria, the powerhouses of our cells, cannot be overstated either. As we age, mitochondrial function declines, leading to less efficient energy production and increased oxidative stress. Enhancing mitochondrial health through nutrition and exercise is another key area to focus on for optimal aging.

Sleep—often underestimated yet incredibly vital—is another cog in the wheel of aging. Quality sleep is essential for cellular repair, cognitive function, and overall wellbeing. Poor sleep accelerates aging, while good sleep habits can help you maintain your youthfulness. Ensuring you have good sleep hygiene is a pillar of extending both lifespan and healthspan.

Social connections, surprisingly, also play a crucial role. Humans are inherently social beings, and isolation can have detrimental effects on both mental and physical health. Multiple studies have shown that strong social ties can actually extend lifespan and improve the quality of life. Never underestimate the power of community in the quest for longevity.

Ah, and don't forget about the mind-body connection. It's becoming increasingly clear that our mental health significantly influences how we age. Chronic stress can accelerate aging by triggering inflammatory responses and shortening telomeres. Techniques like mindfulness and meditation can go a long way in mitigating these effects, bringing harmony to both mind and body.

Let's not ignore the role of lifestyle choices. From what we eat to how active we are, these choices shape our aging process. Embracing a diet rich in whole foods, engaging in regular physical activity, and practicing stress management can collectively slow down aging, enhance vitality, and improve longevity.

Hormonal changes are also a significant part of the aging process. As we age, levels of key hormones like estrogen, testosterone, and growth hormone decline. This can lead to various age-related changes, such as decreased muscle mass, reduced bone density, and altered metabolism. However, there are strategies to mitigate these effects, from dietary adjustments to resistance training exercises that help maintain muscle mass and bone health.

While it might sound like aging is an inevitable decline, that's far from the whole truth. By understanding the underlying mechanisms of aging, we empower ourselves to take actions that promote a longer, healthier life. The power is in your hands to influence many of the variables that affect aging.

What's compelling is how interconnected these aspects of aging are. For instance, a nutrient-dense diet doesn't just fight oxidative stress; it also supports mitochondrial function and hormonal balance. Regular exercise doesn't just keep you fit; it also combats inflammaging and promotes better sleep. Each positive choice you make creates a ripple effect, influencing multiple facets of your health and wellbeing.

Understanding aging isn't about fearing it—it's about embracing it with wisdom and proactive choices. Every glass of water you drink, every evening walk you take, each healthy relationship you nurture—these are all investments in your future self. Remember, aging gracefully isn't about striving for eternal youth; it's about living life fully, with vitality and purpose at every stage.

In unraveling the science of aging, we're not merely looking to add years to our lives but to enhance the quality of those years. By integrating knowledge from genetics, nutrition, physical activity, mental health, and social connections, we can create a holistic approach to aging. This way, every year becomes a new opportunity to live well, laugh often, and love deeply.

So, as you journey through the rest of this book, keep one thing in mind: Aging is not the enemy. It is the natural progression of life, an adventure filled with opportunities to refine, redefine, and reinvent yourself. By understanding and embracing the science of aging, you'll find the keys to not just a longer life, but a life brimming with health, joy, and fulfillment.

Key Longevity Biomarkers

Let's delve into the fascinating world of key longevity biomarkers. These small yet mighty indicators offer a glimpse into our biological age, helping us track and ultimately optimize our journey toward a longer, healthier life. When it comes to promoting longevity, stepping beyond the realm of general advice is essential; understanding these biomarkers takes us deeper, providing personalized insights into our unique aging process.

First, let's talk about *telomeres*. Telomeres are the protective caps at the end of our DNA strands. Think of them like the plastic tips on your shoelaces that keep the ends from fraying. Every time our cells divide, these telomeres get shorter. Once they become too short, the cell can no longer divide, leading to aging and age-related diseases. Studies have shown that longer telomeres are associated with longer life spans. Several lifestyle choices—like reducing stress, adopting a balanced diet, and engaging in regular physical activity—can actually help maintain telomere length.

Inflammation is another critical marker to consider. Chronic inflammation is a well-known contributor to various diseases, including heart disease, diabetes, and even cancer. Specifically, markers like C-reactive protein (CRP) and interleukin-6 (IL-6) can provide insights into the inflammatory status of your body. Keeping these levels in check through diet, exercise, and mindfulness can pave the way for a healthier, longer life.

Hormonal balance also plays a pivotal role. Hormones like cortisol, insulin, and sex hormones (like estrogen and testosterone) can significantly affect how we age. For instance, consistently high levels of cortisol, often called the "stress hormone," can accelerate aging and deteriorate immune function. Meanwhile, insulin resistance can lead to metabolic syndrome, another aging accelerator. Monitoring these hormones offers actionable data on how well your body is managing stress and metabolism—two key areas that influence longevity.

Blood glucose levels are another crucial biomarker. High blood sugar levels can cause damage to our blood vessels, leading to cardiovascular disease, kidney damage, and even cognitive decline. Monitoring fasting glucose and HbA1c levels offers a clear picture of how well your body manages sugar, and by extension, how effectively it's aging. Maintaining balanced blood glucose levels through dietary choices and physical activity is fundamental to longevity.

The health of your gut microbiome is increasingly recognized as another significant biomarker for longevity. Our gut is home to trillions of bacteria which play essential roles in our digestion, immune function, and even our mood. Dysbiosis, or an imbalance of these gut bacteria, can lead to chronic diseases and accelerate the aging process. Fostering a healthy gut microbiome through a diet rich in fiber and fermented foods can significantly enhance your healthspan.

Then, there's heart health, often measured through biomarkers like cholesterol and triglyceride levels. Specifically, maintaining a healthy ratio of HDL (good cholesterol) to LDL (bad cholesterol) is vital for cardiovascular health. Similarly, keeping an eye on triglycerides, or fatty acids in the blood, can provide insights into your metabolic health. Elevated levels can signal a higher risk of heart disease, but these can be managed through diet, exercise, and sometimes medication.

Oxidative stress is another area worth monitoring. Our bodies generate free radicals as a byproduct of normal metabolism, but too many of these can damage cells and accelerate aging. Biomarkers like malondialdehyde (MDA) and 8-hydroxydeoxyguanosine (8-OHdG) can indicate levels of oxidative damage. Incorporating antioxidant-rich foods into your diet helps neutralize free radicals and lower oxidative stress.

Finally, genetic markers can give us a predictive edge. While we can't change our genetic makeup, understanding certain genetic markers can help us tailor our lifestyle choices to better align with our biological predispositions. For instance, some people might be genetically predisposed to higher levels of inflammation or oxidative stress. Knowing this, they can take specific preventative measures to counteract these risks.

So, why focus on these biomarkers? Because they offer a tangible, measurable way of assessing where we stand in our health and longevity journey. Instead of guessing, we're using science to guide us. This knowledge empowers us to make informed decisions that can significantly impact not just the length of our lives, but the quality as well.

As you start to incorporate these insights into your daily routine, remember that small, consistent changes often yield the most significant results. Maintaining healthy levels of these biomarkers isn't about making drastic changes overnight. It's about creating sustainable habits that fit seamlessly into your lifestyle.

In conclusion, the key longevity biomarkers—telomere length, inflammation markers, hormonal balance, glucose levels, gut health, heart health, oxidative stress, and genetic markers—serve as vital signposts on our path to a longer, healthier life. By regularly monitoring and optimizing these markers, we arm ourselves with the knowledge needed to make meaningful changes, steering our lives toward enhanced longevity and well-being.

Embrace the science, trust your journey, and remember that every step you take towards understanding and optimizing these biomarkers is a step towards a richer, more vibrant life.

Chapter 2:
Nutrition for a Long Life

E ating isn't just about fueling our bodies; it's about nourishing our souls and crafting a life of vitality. Imagine your body as a garden. The foods you choose are the seeds you plant, and the care you give them determines how lush and resilient your garden becomes. Whole foods, brimming with the earth's natural power, act as the building blocks of a healthy, long life. They're rich in the nutrients our bodies crave. Superfoods add an extra punch, bringing a wealth of antioxidants and anti-inflammatory nutrients that combat the wear and tear of daily living. And let's not overlook the magic of fasting, which can reset and rejuvenate, giving your body the break it needs to repair and thrive. The journey to longevity begins on your plate, and with each mindful bite, you're making an investment in a vibrant future.

The Power of Whole Foods

The role of nutrition in extending our lifespan can't be overstated, and it all begins with the quality and type of food we consume. At the heart of any nutritional strategy for longevity lies the concept of whole foods. Let's dive into why whole foods are a cornerstone of a healthy diet and how they can help pave the way for a longer, more vibrant life.

Whole foods are essentially foods that are as close to their natural form as possible. Think fresh fruits and vegetables, whole grains, legumes, nuts, seeds, and unprocessed animal products. These foods are packed with essential nutrients that our bodies crave—vitamins, minerals, fiber, and phytochemicals—that work synergistically to promote health and ward off disease.

Why are whole foods so powerful? It's because they're nature's perfect package. For instance, when you eat an apple, you're not just getting vitamin C; you're also consuming fiber, various antioxidants, and a host of other compounds that work together to benefit your body. The same cannot be said for many processed foods that often strip away these beneficial elements, leaving behind empty calories.

Whole foods also help in maintaining a balanced weight—a key factor in longevity. Processed foods often contain unhealthy fats, added sugars, and a slew of artificial additives that can lead to weight gain and metabolic issues. In contrast, whole foods are generally lower in calories and higher in nutrients, helping you feel full and satisfied without overeating.

Consider the impact on your digestive system. The fiber found in whole foods is crucial for maintaining a healthy gut microbiome. A balanced microbiome supports digestion, boosts the immune system, and may even affect mood and mental health. Inadequate fiber intake, commonly seen in diets high in processed foods, can lead to digestive problems and inflammatory diseases.

Studies have consistently shown that individuals who consume diets rich in whole foods tend to have lower rates of chronic diseases such as heart disease, diabetes, and cancer. These diseases are often the result of long-term damage caused by poor nutrition and inflammation. By embracing whole foods, you give your body the tools it needs to repair and protect itself.

Let's talk about some practical ways to integrate more whole foods into your diet. Start your day with a hearty bowl of oatmeal topped with fresh berries and nuts, rather than a sugary cereal. For lunch, opt for a colorful salad loaded with different vegetables, legumes, and a healthy dressing. These small changes can make a huge difference over time.

Incorporating whole foods doesn't mean you have to give up flavor or satisfaction. Whole foods are remarkably diverse and can be prepared in countless delicious ways. Roasted vegetables, flavorful stews, fresh fruit salads, and an array of whole grains can elevate your meals while nourishing your body.

Shopping for whole foods can be an enjoyable experience as well. Farmers' markets and local grocery stores often provide a plethora of seasonal produce, allowing you to connect with your food more deeply. Seasonal eating not only ensures you get the freshest produce but also supports local farmers and reduces your carbon footprint.

Another key advantage of whole foods is their role in managing blood sugar levels. Unlike refined sugars and carbohydrates, whole foods are digested more slowly, providing a steady release of energy. This can help in preventing the blood sugar spikes and crashes that are common with processed foods, thereby reducing the risk of developing type 2 diabetes.

Let's not forget about hydration. Whole foods, especially fruits and vegetables, have high water content that contributes to your daily hydration needs. Staying well-hydrated is crucial for maintaining bodily functions, improving skin health, and even aiding in cognitive functions.

Moreover, whole foods are inherently anti-inflammatory. Chronic inflammation is a silent killer, often contributing to the development of debilitating diseases. Foods like leafy greens, fatty fish, and berries are packed with anti-inflammatory compounds. By choosing these over processed alternatives, you're not just nourishing your body; you're actively fighting inflammation.

Whole foods also help in maintaining hormonal balance. Nutrient-dense foods provide the necessary vitamins and minerals that help regulate hormones. This is particularly important for aging, as hormonal imbalances can lead to a variety of health issues including weight gain, fatigue, and mood swings.

Another significant aspect to consider is sustainability. Whole foods generally have a smaller environmental footprint compared to their processed counterparts. By consuming more plant-based whole foods, you contribute to a more sustainable food system, which is increasingly important in our fight against climate change.

Incorporating more whole foods doesn't have to be a daunting task. Begin by making simple swaps in your daily meals. Replace processed snacks with fresh fruit or a handful of nuts. Choose whole grain bread over white bread. Small, consistent changes are often the most sustainable and impactful.

Additionally, whole foods can be a joy to cook with. Discover new recipes and cooking techniques that focus on using fresh, unprocessed ingredients. This can rekindle your relationship with food, turning meal preparation into an enjoyable and meditative practice.

The community aspect of food shouldn't be overlooked either. Preparing and sharing whole food-based meals with loved ones can strengthen social bonds and promote a culture of health and wellness. These social connections are essential for mental and emotional well-being, adding another layer to the benefits of whole foods.

Remember, the journey to longevity and optimal health is a holistic one, consisting of many small, deliberate choices. Embracing the power of whole foods is a foundational step, setting the stage for a life that is not just longer, but richer in vitality, joy, and well-being.

Giving your body what it needs through whole foods is one of the most loving actions you can take. The benefits extend far beyond mere nutrition—they permeate every aspect of your physical, mental, and emotional health. So, take the first step today. Your future self will thank you.

Superfoods and Their Benefits

When it comes to adding years to your life and life to your years, superfoods pack an incredible punch. These nutrient-dense foods bring a host of benefits that can give you the energy of your youth while fortifying your body against the wear and tear of aging. Think of the vibrant color of blueberries, the rich texture of avocados, and the boldness of dark leafy greens. They're more than just foods; they're nature's multivitamins. The antioxidants in these powerhouse foods combat oxidative stress, while anti-inflammatory properties curtail chronic diseases. Picture your body rejoicing at each bite, cells rejuvenating and energy levels soaring. Incorporating these superfoods into your diet is like planting seeds for a more prosperous and enduring life ahead. You'll not only feel the difference but radiate health from the inside out. So, let your plate be a vibrant palette, painting the portrait of a long, healthy, and fulfilled life.

Antioxidant-Rich Foods ... Embarking on a journey toward a longer and healthier life, antioxidant-rich foods are your trusty companions. These mighty morsels, abundant in vibrant colors and tantalizing flavors, go beyond mere sustenance. They hold the keys to combating oxidative stress, which plays a significant role in the aging process. Incorporating these foods into your daily diet can be transformative, making each meal a step toward a more youthful you.

Oxidative stress occurs when there's an imbalance between free radicals and antioxidants in your body. Free radicals are unstable molecules that can cause cell damage, eventually leading to chronic diseases and aging. Think of them as tiny villains wreaking havoc within your cells. But we're not defenseless in this battle; antioxidants are the heroes that neutralize these free radicals, maintaining cellular health and vitality.

Imagine biting into a juicy blueberry and savoring not just its sweet taste, but also its wealth of antioxidants. Blueberries, along with other berries like strawberries and raspberries, are powerhouses when it comes to protecting your cells. They're packed with anthocyanins, a type of antioxidant responsible for their rich, deep colors. So next time you sprinkle some berries on your yogurt or blend them into a smoothie, remember, you're doing much more than just pleasing your taste buds.

The vibrant hues of fruits and vegetables are more than just eye candy—they're a sign of nutrient density. Carrots with their bright orange, spinach with its lush green, and tomatoes with their vivid red, are brimming with antioxidants like beta-carotene, lutein, and lycopene. These compounds have been shown to protect against various forms of cancer, improve skin health, and even boost your immune system. Eating the rainbow isn't just a catchy phrase; it's a simple yet powerful guideline for ensuring you're getting a broad spectrum of protective antioxidants.

Holy guacamole! Avocados deserve a special mention. Not only are they creamy and delicious, but they're also loaded with glutathione, a potent antioxidant that supports liver health and detoxification processes. Toss it in a salad or spread it on toast—avocados are a versatile, nutrient-rich addition to any meal.

Don't forget about your spice rack. Turmeric, ginger, and cinnamon aren't just flavor enhancers; they're antioxidant goldmines. Curcumin, the active compound in turmeric, has been studied extensively for its anti-inflammatory and antioxidant properties. Similarly, ginger is celebrated for its medicinal traits, including combating oxidative stress. Even a simple act of spicing up your dish can impart significant health benefits.

Nuts and seeds are another fantastic source of antioxidants. Almonds, walnuts, chia seeds, and flaxseeds offer a wonderful crunch while providing essential nutrients and antioxidants like vitamin E and selenium. These nutrients are known to repair damaged cells and reduce the risk of heart disease. A handful of nuts not only keeps the midday hunger at bay but also arms your body with tools to fight cellular damage.

Green tea is often hailed as a miracle drink, and for good reason. It's loaded with catechins, particularly epigallocatechin gallate (EGCG), an antioxidant that has powerful effects on health. Regular consumption of green tea has been linked to improved brain function, fat loss, and reduced risk of some cancers. Sipping on this ancient brew can be a simple yet profoundly beneficial habit.

Then there are the dark, leafy greens—kale, spinach, and Swiss chard. These nutrient-rich vegetables are packed with antioxidants like lutein and zeaxanthin, which support eye health and lower the risk of macular degeneration. They're also fantastic sources of vitamins A, C, and K. Toss them in your salad, blend them into a smoothie, or sauté them for a nutrient-packed side dish.

Let's talk legumes. Beans, lentils, and chickpeas aren't just for soups and stews; they're reservoirs of antioxidants and fiber. Red kidney beans, in particular, have an incredibly high antioxidant content, rivaling even some berries. Incorporating these into your meals can aid in digestion, stabilize blood sugar levels, and promote a healthier gut.

Citrus fruits like oranges, lemons, and grapefruits are brimming with vitamin C, a superstar antioxidant. Vitamin C boosts your immune system, enhances skin health, and aids in the repair of body tissues. Whether squeezed into a refreshing juice or peeled for a midday snack, citrus fruits are a zesty way to infuse your diet with vital nutrients.

Cruciferous vegetables such as broccoli, Brussels sprouts, and cauliflower are not to be overlooked. They contain sulforaphane, an antioxidant that turns on the detoxifying enzymes in the body. These vegetables are also high in fiber, vitamins, and minerals, making them an excellent addition to your diet for both their nutritional and protective benefits.

Each of these foods, with their unique profiles of antioxidants, contributes to a balanced diet that fights off aging at the cellular level. As you build your meals, think of each ingredient as more than just calories—it's an investment in your longevity. By diversifying your diet with a range of antioxidant-rich foods, you create a robust defense system against the wear and tear of life.

As a health-conscious individual looking to optimize your well-being, understanding the power of antioxidant-rich foods can be a game changer. The beauty of these foods lies in their accessibility and versatility. They're not exotic items that require a trek to a specialty store; they're everyday ingredients that you can begin incorporating into your diet right now. The real magic happens when these diverse nutrients come together to create a symphony of health benefits.

Consider making meal preparation a joyful and mindful practice, focusing on integrating a variety of colors, textures, and flavors that antioxidant-rich foods offer. By doing so, you not only nourish your body but also engage your senses in a way that promotes overall well-being. Remember, health is holistic—all parts of you deserve the tender, loving care that comes from both nutritious food and joyful eating experiences.

The journey to longevity and vibrant health is paved with the choices we make daily. Antioxidant-rich foods offer a simple yet profound way to protect our bodies from the inside out. By making them a staple in your diet, you empower yourself with one of nature's most potent tools for preserving health and extending lifespan.

In the grand scheme of things, it's these small, consistent choices that add up to significant differences. Imagine your cells smiling with each bite of an antioxidant-rich berry or each sip of a green tea. It's these moments that stitch together a life of wellness and longevity, weaving a tapestry of health that can stand the test of time.

Anti-Inflammatory Nutrients play a crucial role in maintaining overall health and extending lifespan. Inflammation is a natural response of the immune system to injury or infection, but chronic inflammation is linked to numerous age-related diseases, including heart disease, diabetes, and Alzheimer's. By incorporating anti-inflammatory nutrients into your diet, you can safeguard your health and boost your longevity.

One of the cornerstones of anti-inflammatory nutrition is omega-3 fatty acids. These powerful fats are found in abundance in fish like salmon, mackerel, and sardines, as well as in plant sources like flaxseeds, chia seeds, and walnuts. Omega-3s have been shown to reduce inflammation at the molecular level, decreasing the production of inflammatory substances called cytokines. Incorporating these foods into your diet a few times a week can make a significant difference.

If you're a fan of spices, you'll be pleased to know that some of your kitchen staples have potent anti-inflammatory properties. Turmeric, for instance, contains curcumin, a compound that has been extensively studied for its ability to reduce inflammation. Adding a dash of turmeric to your meals or enjoying a turmeric latte can be a delicious way to enhance your health. Ginger is another spice that offers anti-inflammatory benefits. Whether you use it in teas, smoothies, or cooking, ginger can help soothe inflammation and improve digestion.

Don't underestimate the power of fruits and vegetables in the fight against chronic inflammation. Berries, especially blueberries, strawberries, and raspberries, are packed with antioxidants that combat oxidative stress and inflammation. Leafy greens like spinach, kale, and Swiss chard are rich in vitamins and minerals that support your body's natural defenses. These foods not only reduce inflammation but also provide a myriad of other health benefits, making them essential components of a longevity-focused diet.

It's not just what you eat but also how you prepare your food that can influence inflammation levels. For instance, cooking methods that involve high temperatures and prolonged cooking times can produce advanced glycation end-products (AGEs), which are linked to increased inflammation. Opting for gentler cooking methods like steaming, poaching, or cooking at lower temperatures can help minimize the formation of AGEs and keep inflammation at bay.

Whole grains are another important group of foods to consider. Unlike refined grains, whole grains retain all parts of the grain, including the bran, germ, and endosperm. This means they are richer in fiber, vitamins, and minerals, all of which play a role in reducing inflammation. Foods like quinoa, brown rice, oatmeal, and whole-wheat products can improve your gut health and reduce inflammation, providing you with sustained energy throughout the day.

Another powerhouse in the realm of anti-inflammatory nutrients is the family of monounsaturated fats. Found in foods like olive oil, avocados, and nuts, these fats help to lower the body's inflammatory response. Olive oil, in particular, contains oleocanthal, a compound that mimics the anti-inflammatory effect of ibuprofen. A drizzle of extra-virgin olive oil on your salad or in your cooking can be both tasty and beneficial for your health.

Polyphenols found in tea and coffee also deserve a shout-out. Green tea, for example, contains a polyphenol called epigallocatechin gallate (EGCG), which has potent anti-inflammatory effects. Similarly, the polyphenols in coffee can help reduce inflammation and protect against chronic diseases. Enjoying these beverages in moderation can be a part of your anti-inflammatory strategy.

Dark chocolate lovers, rejoice! Dark chocolate with a high cocoa content (70% or more) is rich in flavonoids, which have anti-inflammatory properties. These compounds can help reduce inflammation and even improve endothelial function, which is crucial for heart health. A small piece of dark chocolate can be a delightful treat that also supports your longevity goals.

Probiotic-rich foods like yogurt, kefir, sauerkraut, and kimchi can also modulate inflammation. The gut microbiome plays a significant role in regulating the immune system and inflammation. By nourishing your gut with probiotics, you can promote the growth of beneficial bacteria, which in turn, helps reduce inflammation and improve overall health.

Lastly, hydration plays a subtle yet essential role in managing inflammation. Drinking enough water helps your body flush out toxins and supports all bodily functions, including the immune system. Proper hydration ensures that your cells function optimally, reducing the likelihood of chronic inflammation.

Incorporating these anti-inflammatory nutrients into your daily routine doesn't have to be complicated. Simple swaps and thoughtful meal planning can make a world of difference. Instead of refined sugars and white bread, opt for fruits, whole grains, and healthy fats. Choose cooking methods that preserve the nutritional integrity of your food, and spice up your meals with turmeric and ginger.

In summary, a diet rich in anti-inflammatory nutrients is one of the most effective ways to promote longevity and protect against age-related diseases. From omega-3 fatty acids and spices like turmeric and ginger, to antioxidant-rich fruits and vegetables, whole grains, monounsaturated fats, and probiotic-rich foods, these dietary components work synergistically to combat inflammation and support overall health. Remember, the journey to a longer, healthier life is paved with small, mindful choices each day. Embrace these anti-inflammatory strategies and watch as they transform not just your diet, but your entire approach to wellness.

The Role of Fasting

Fasting isn't just a trend; it's been part of human culture for centuries, anchored in a multitude of religious and spiritual practices. But it's more than just skipping meals for soul-searching—fasting carries a host of physical benefits that modern science is just beginning to fully understand. Let's dive into why fasting can be a game-changer for your health and longevity.

For starters, let's talk about autophagy. It's a natural cellular process that involves the breakdown and recycling of damaged cellular components. Think of it as your body's internal housekeeping service, cleaning out the clutter that can slow you down. Fasting triggers autophagy, allowing your cells to rejuvenate themselves, which plays a crucial role in longevity. Imagine hitting the reset button on a cluttered room and finding all the extra space you never knew you had—fasting does exactly that for your cells.

Another remarkable benefit is fasting's effect on insulin sensitivity. We often hear about how a Western diet high in refined sugars and processed foods can lead to insulin resistance, setting the stage for type 2 diabetes and other chronic illnesses. When you fast, though, your body gets a break from the continuous influx of glucose, allowing it to reset its insulin sensitivity. This can lead to more stable blood sugar levels, reduced risk of diabetes, and an overall improvement in metabolic health.

Of course, it's essential to mention the potential for weight management. For those looking to shed a few pounds or maintain a healthy weight, fasting can act as a powerful tool. By narrowing your eating window, whether it's through intermittent fasting or another method, you naturally reduce your calorie intake without the need to meticulously count each morsel of food. Fasting can simplify your eating habits, making it easier to manage your weight in the long term.

But the benefits aren't just physical; they extend to the brain as well. Cognitive health is a significant concern as we age, with risks of neurodegenerative conditions like Alzheimer's and Parkinson's. There's promising research suggesting that fasting can enhance brain function and promote the production of brain-derived neurotrophic factor (BDNF). This protein supports the survival and growth of neurons, essentially acting as a fertilizer for your brain cells. Clearer thinking, improved memory, and better focus—these are the cognitive perks that fasting can offer.

Now, before you jump headfirst into a fasting regimen, it's crucial to understand that it's not a one-size-fits-all approach. There are various methods to consider. Intermittent fasting, for example, is one of the most popular forms. It involves cycling between periods of eating and fasting, such as the 16/8 method, where you fast for 16 hours and eat during an 8-hour window. The 5:2 method, another common variant, involves eating normally for five days and significantly reducing calorie intake for two non-consecutive days.

Extended fasting, which involves going without food for 24 hours or more, can also offer profound benefits but requires more caution and preparation. It's not something you should dive into without understanding its impact on your body and consulting with a healthcare professional, especially if you have underlying health conditions.

How you break your fast is equally vital. The first meal after a fasting period should be balanced and nutrient-rich, avoiding overly processed foods and sugars. It's like waking up your digestive system gently instead of shocking it into submission. A meal full of whole foods—like lean proteins, healthy fats, and fresh vegetables—will help you reap the full benefits of your fasting period and set the tone for the rest of your eating window.

Moreover, hydration is crucial during fasting periods. While you're abstaining from food, it's important to drink plenty of water. Some fasting methods even allow for beverages like herbal teas, black coffee, or bone broth. Staying hydrated helps to manage hunger and supports various bodily functions, making your fasting experience more comfortable.

Let's not forget the mind-body connection here. Fasting isn't just a physical act; it often involves a degree of mental discipline. It can teach you a lot about your eating patterns and emotional triggers. When you fast, you become more aware of when you eat out of boredom, stress, or habit rather than true hunger. This knowledge can be empowering, leading to a healthier relationship with food.

On another note, community can play a role in your fasting journey as well. Engaging in fasting with a group or sharing experiences with others can provide encouragement, shared tips, and motivation. It can become a social occasion, turning fasting into a collective lifestyle change rather than a solitary experience.

So, with all these benefits, why isn't everyone fasting? Well, the main obstacles are often misconceptions and a lack of understanding. Some people worry they'll feel weak, irritable, or overly hungry. True, the initial stages can be challenging, but as your body adapts, many find that their energy levels stabilize and hunger pangs diminish. The key is to start slow, listen to your body, and adjust as needed.

It's also important to note that fasting isn't for everyone. Pregnant or breastfeeding women, individuals with a history of eating disorders, and anyone with certain health conditions should approach fasting with extra caution. Always consult a healthcare provider before starting a new fasting regimen to ensure it's a safe choice for you.

In essence, fasting is more than a dietary tweak—it's a holistic tool with the potential to transform your physical health, mental clarity, and emotional well-being. Imagine feeling lighter, both in body and mind, more focused, and in control of your health. That's the real magic of fasting. By embracing this practice, you're not just choosing a healthier lifestyle; you're investing in your future self. You're gifting yourself the potential for a longer, healthier, and more vibrant life. Isn't that a journey worth embarking on?

Chapter 3:
Exercise and Physical Activity

We've all heard it: exercise is essential for a healthy life. But let's be real—it's not just about hitting the gym or pounding the pavement. It's about moving your body in ways that feel good and make you stronger, more resilient, and brimming with vitality. Physical activity is your passport to longevity. It invigorates your muscles, boosts your cardiovascular system, and even sharpens your cognitive functions. Whether you prefer a brisk walk, a yoga flow, or a heart-pumping HIIT session, what matters is consistency and joy in movement. Make it social, make it fun. Because when you find an exercise routine that makes you light up inside, you're not just adding years to your life; you're investing in quality years. In this chapter, we'll explore various exercise modes and uncover how each can uniquely contribute to your golden years.

The Best Exercises for Longevity

You don't need to be an elite athlete to experience the remarkable benefits of exercise for longevity. The best exercises for extending your lifespan and enhancing your quality of life combine strength training, cardiovascular workouts, flexibility exercises, and balance activities. Incorporating a mix of these into your weekly routine can work wonders. Imagine building muscle with regular strength training sessions, invigorating your heart with a brisk run, cycling, or swimming, and improving your flexibility and balance with yoga or tai chi. These activities not only ward off frailty but also keep your mind sharp and your mood elevated. It's not about pushing yourself to your limits; it's about finding the right balance that keeps you moving and growing, mentally and physically, as the years go by. Through consistent, varied exercise, you unlock the potential to live a longer, more vibrant life.

Strength Training is not just for bodybuilders or athletes; it's an essential component for anyone looking to enhance their health and longevity. You might wonder why lifting weights could be relevant to living longer. The truth is, the benefits of strength training extend far beyond building muscle. Incorporating regular strength training into your life can be transformative, affecting everything from your metabolic rate to your cognitive function. When we focus on longevity, we're not just talking about adding years to your life but also life to your years.

One of the most significant perks of strength training is its impact on your metabolic health. By increasing muscle mass, you improve your body's ability to burn calories more efficiently. This helps maintain a healthy weight and can prevent metabolic disorders like type 2 diabetes. Muscle tissue is metabolically active, meaning it burns more calories at rest compared to fat tissue. The more muscle you have, the more energy your body expends, even when you're not working out. This can be a game-changer for weight management, especially as you age.

Another noteworthy advantage is strength training's role in enhancing bone density. Osteoporosis and fractures are common concerns as we get older. Weight-bearing exercises, including weight lifting and resistance training, stimulate bone growth and increase bone density. This makes bones stronger and reduces the risk of fractures. In essence, strength training can literally help you stand stronger, adding a layer of resilience to your body as you age.

But let's not forget about the role of strength training in functional fitness. Functional fitness refers to the ability to perform everyday activities with ease. Think about carrying groceries, climbing stairs, or even playing with your grandchildren. Strength training improves muscle strength and endurance, making these daily tasks less strenuous. Enhanced functional fitness contributes to an overall better quality of life, which is a cornerstone of longevity.

There's also a profound connection between strength training and mental health. Exercise in general releases endorphins, which are natural mood lifters. But strength training, in particular, has been found to reduce symptoms of anxiety and depression. Completing a challenging workout provides a sense of accomplishment, which can boost your confidence and improve your overall outlook on life. Moreover, the focus required during strength training offers a form of mindfulness, grounding you in the present moment and reducing stress levels.

Don't underestimate the social benefits of strength training either. Whether you're hitting the gym, attending a fitness class, or working out with a friend, the social interactions can be incredibly enriching. Building a sense of community and establishing a support network can improve adherence to your fitness regime. The camaraderie found in group workout settings can enhance your motivation, making it easier to maintain a consistent exercise routine.

When it comes to cognitive function, strength training offers surprising benefits. Studies suggest that resistance exercises can improve memory, attention, and information processing. The increased blood flow to the brain during physical activity contributes to maintaining and even enhancing cognitive functions. There's a growing body of evidence indicating that staying physically strong correlates with mental fortitude, reducing the risk of cognitive decline in later years.

So, how do you get started with strength training if it's new to you? Initially, focus on learning proper form and technique. Poor form can lead to injuries, counteracting all the benefits you're aiming for. It might be worthwhile to consult a fitness professional or personal trainer who can guide you through the basics. Start with lighter weights and gradually increase the intensity as your strength builds. Consistency is key, so aim for at least two to three strength training sessions per week.

Variety is another essential aspect. Incorporate different types of resistance exercises to target various muscle groups. This not only ensures balanced muscle development but also keeps your workouts interesting. Free weights, machines, body-weight exercises, and resistance bands all have their place in a well-rounded strength training regimen. Each type offers unique advantages, and rotating through different methods can help prevent plateaus.

Recovery is just as important as the workouts themselves. Giving your muscles time to repair and grow is crucial for progress. Incorporate rest days into your routine and pay attention to your body's signals. Sufficient sleep, proper nutrition, and hydration also play significant roles in recovery. Don't hesitate to consult healthcare providers or fitness experts if you're unsure about any aspect of your strength training journey.

Some people worry about bulking up too much, but it's essential to understand that building excessive muscle mass usually requires a very specific and intense training regime alongside a specialized diet. For the average person, strength training will help create a lean, toned physique, not transform you into a bodybuilder. Most importantly, it builds the strength and resilience needed for a long, healthy life.

In conclusion, strength training is a versatile and indispensable tool in your longevity toolkit. From metabolic health and bone density to functional fitness and mental well-being, its benefits are extensive and profound. By embracing resistance exercises, you're investing in a future where you not only live longer but thrive with vitality, strength, and an indomitable spirit. Make strength training a regular part of your lifestyle and you'll find yourself better equipped to enjoy every moment of your life with vigor and enthusiasm.

Cardiovascular Health is a cornerstone of overall well-being and longevity. Your heart, the unassuming powerhouse in your chest, quietly supports every aspect of your life. While we often take it for granted until something goes awry, safeguarding our cardiovascular health is paramount.

The simplest way to think about cardiovascular health is to view it as the engine behind your body's performance. Just like any engine, it needs proper care and maintenance. Neglecting it isn't really an option if you're aiming for a long and vibrant life. But fear not, taking steps to improve your cardiovascular health isn't some Herculean task; it's about making smarter, daily choices.

So, where do we begin? Exercise, of course. Regular aerobic activities such as walking, jogging, swimming, or even dancing can significantly improve your heart's efficiency. The magic number here is at least 150 minutes of moderate-intensity exercise per week. If you're short on time, aim for 75 minutes of high-intensity workouts. Exercise helps lower blood pressure, reduces bad cholesterol, and raises good cholesterol. But let's not forget the joy factor – finding an activity you love will make it an enduring part of your life.

Remember, it's not about torturing yourself with activities you hate. Rather, it's about integrating physical movements you enjoy. A brisk morning walk can be just as beneficial as a high-intensity cardio session, as long as you're consistent. Think of your daily stroll as a love letter to your heart.

Diet plays an equally vital role in maintaining cardiovascular health. Embrace a diet rich in whole foods, including fruits, vegetables, whole grains, nuts, and seeds. Omega-3 fatty acids, found in fish like salmon and mackerel, are particularly heart-friendly. They help reduce triglycerides, lower blood pressure, and prevent irregular heartbeats. Want a simpler approach? Think of your plate as a colorful palette where greens, reds, and purples take center stage. The brighter and more varied the colors, the better for your heart.

Another aspect that's crucial yet often overlooked is hydration. Proper hydration ensures that blood volume is maintained, making it easier for your heart to pump blood. Aim for at least eight cups of water a day, but adjust according to your activity level and climate. Remember, caffeinated beverages and alcohol can dehydrate you, so balance them out with extra water.

Processed foods and unhealthy fats are your heart's nemesis. Trans fats, commonly found in fried foods, baked goods, and snacks, should be avoided like the plague. They not only raise your bad cholesterol but also lower your good cholesterol. Next time you're grocery shopping, be an ingredient detective. Check labels and avoid anything that lists hydrogenated oils. Instead, focus on good fats from sources like avocados, olive oil, and nuts, which help to keep your arteries flexible and resilient.

Stress is another silent saboteur of cardiovascular health. When you're stressed, your body releases hormones like adrenaline and cortisol, which make your heart work harder. Chronic stress can lead to high blood pressure, a major risk factor for heart disease. Learning stress management techniques such as mindfulness, deep breathing, or even taking short breaks throughout the day can make a huge difference.

Let's not underestimate the power of laughter and joy. Engaging in activities that make you happy can lower your stress hormones, decrease inflammation, and increase your levels of good cholesterol. Whether it's spending time with loved ones, indulging in hobbies, or simply watching a funny movie, joy and laughter truly are the best medicine.

Smoking is one habit you can't afford to maintain if you're serious about cardiovascular health. The harmful chemicals in tobacco damage your blood vessels and heart, leading to an increased risk of atherosclerosis, heart attack, and stroke. Quitting smoking, on the other hand, can lower your heart disease risk significantly in just one year.

Alcohol consumption is another area where moderation is key. While a glass of red wine here and there can be beneficial thanks to its antioxidant properties, excessive drinking is detrimental. Too much alcohol can elevate blood pressure, contribute to obesity, and lead to heart failure. If you drink, do so in moderation.

Sleep is the often-neglected pillar of cardiovascular health. Poor sleep quality and short sleep durations are linked with increased risk for cardiovascular diseases. Your body uses sleep time to repair itself, including your heart and blood vessels. Aim for at least 7-9 hours of quality sleep each night. Maintain a consistent sleep schedule and create a restful environment to ensure you're getting the most out of your slumber.

Don't forget the social element. Strong social connections can reduce stress and promote a sense of well-being, both of which are beneficial for your heart. People who have satisfying social ties are shown to have lower blood pressure, better heart rates, and more robust immune systems. So, spend time with people who lift you up, and don't shy away from forming new connections. Your heart will thank you!

Finally, let's discuss the importance of regular check-ups. Annual health screenings can catch potential issues early, allowing for timely intervention. Monitoring your blood pressure, cholesterol levels, and blood sugar can help you keep tabs on your heart health and make necessary adjustments. Knowledge is power, and in this case, it's the power to live healthier, longer.

In summary, a heart-healthy lifestyle doesn't require drastic measures. It's about making consistent, thoughtful choices every day. Exercise regularly, eat a balanced diet, stay hydrated, manage stress, get enough sleep, and embrace social connections. Your heart is more than just an organ; it's the rhythm of your life. Treat it well, and it will reward you with years of vitality and joy.

Flexibility and Balance

Flexibility and balance are often overlooked components of a well-rounded fitness regimen, yet they are absolutely essential for longevity and overall well-being. As we age, our muscles and joints can lose their elasticity, leading to stiffness, discomfort, and a higher risk of injury. Meanwhile, balance becomes increasingly crucial to prevent falls and maintain independence. By focusing on these aspects of physical health, you're not just adding years to your life, but life to your years. Let's dive into why these often-neglected practices are pivotal for long-term health and quality of life.

When we think about physical fitness, the mind often drifts to images of weightlifting and high-intensity interval training. While these are important, flexibility and balance offer subtle yet profound benefits that can transform how you move and feel daily. Picture a world where you can bend, twist, and turn without strain—where every movement seems fluid and effortless. That world is attainable through consistent flexibility and balance training.

Stretching is the cornerstone of improving flexibility. Not only does it help in elongating muscles, but it also enhances blood flow, promotes muscle recovery, and reduces stress. Imagine your muscles as rubber bands: over time, if they're not stretched properly, they become brittle and more prone to snapping. Regular stretching routines can keep your muscles supple and resilient, helping you maintain a full range of motion and reducing the risk of injuries.

You don't need to be a yoga master to reap the benefits of stretching. Simple activities like reaching for your toes, extending your arms overhead, and performing spinal twists can significantly enhance your flexibility. Incorporate these movements into your daily routine, perhaps even multiple times a day. The key here is consistency, not intensity. Gentle, sustained stretches that take you just a little beyond your comfort zone are often the most effective.

Balance, on the other hand, demands a different kind of attention. While stretching keeps us limber, balance training ensures that we can navigate our environment with ease and confidence. Think of balance as the unsung hero behind every step you take and every move you make. It allows you to stand on one leg, walk on uneven surfaces, and recover from potential trips.

Exercises like standing on one foot, walking heel to toe, and practicing tai chi are exceptionally beneficial for enhancing balance. Even something as simple as standing while putting on your socks can serve as an impromptu balance exercise. The beauty of balance training lies in its adaptability; you can integrate these exercises into your daily life without needing specialized equipment or extensive time commitments.

For many, yoga and Pilates are game-changers that fuse both flexibility and balance into cohesive practice. These disciplines offer more than just physical benefits; they also cultivate a sense of mental calm and focus. The slow, deliberate movements and deep breathing exercises inherent in yoga and Pilates encourage mindfulness and stress reduction, promoting mental well-being alongside physical health.

Beyond traditional exercises, incorporating more movement into your daily routine can drastically improve both your flexibility and balance. Think about taking the stairs instead of the elevator, choosing to walk or cycle for short trips, or even dancing in your living room. Every bit of movement counts and contributes to a more agile, balanced you.

Incorporating flexibility and balance into your regimen doesn't mean abandoning other forms of exercise. Instead, see it as a complementary practice that enhances your overall fitness. Strength training, cardio, and flexibility and balance training can coexist harmoniously, each contributing in unique ways to your health and longevity.

Perhaps one of the most compelling reasons to prioritize flexibility and balance is the impact on daily living activities. Simple tasks that we often take for granted—bending down to pick something up, reaching for an item on a high shelf, or quickly changing direction while walking—become easier and safer. When your body moves smoothly and your balance is on point, mundane tasks turn into effortless actions.

Moreover, good balance and flexibility reduce the likelihood of falls, which are a significant concern as we age. Falls can lead to severe injuries, prolonged recovery periods, and diminished quality of life. By strengthening your body's ability to maintain equilibrium and move efficiently, you can dramatically reduce this risk, thereby safeguarding your autonomy and outdoor activity levels.

To sum it up, flexibility and balance are not just supplementary aspects of fitness; they are foundational. They can enhance your ability to perform other exercises more effectively and with less risk of injury.

They improve posture, reduce muscle tension, and support better biomechanics, leading to more fluid and harmonious movement patterns.

Incorporating flexibility and balance exercises into your lifestyle doesn't require a significant time investment. Even just a few minutes daily dedicated to stretching and balance exercises can make a substantial difference. Start small, and gradually increase the duration and complexity of your exercises as your body adapts and strengthens.

Your journey towards improved flexibility and balance is a personal one. It may be filled with small victories and occasional setbacks, but each step forward brings you closer to a more agile, balanced, and vital self. Remember, it's not about achieving perfection but about making consistent, mindful progress. Your body, now and in the future, will thank you for the commitment.

Ultimately, the goal is to create a life rich in movement and vitality. By paying attention to flexibility and balance today, you're sowing the seeds for a tomorrow filled with grace, strength, and freedom. So, stretch a bit further, stand a bit taller, and embrace the myriad ways your body can move through the world. The benefits will be lifelong, enriching every other aspect of your physical and mental health on this incredible journey towards longevity and wellness.

Chapter 4:
The Role of Mental Health

Mental health isn't just the absence of mental illness; it's the wellspring of a vibrant, fulfilling life. When our minds are free from the clutches of chronic stress, anxiety, and depression, we unlock a vast reservoir of energy and resilience that cascades through every facet of our being. A sound mind creates a domino effect, reinforcing our body's ability to fend off diseases and age gracefully. Think of your mental health like a cornerstone, anchoring the myriad pillars of your well-being. Without it, the edifice of health falters, no matter how robust other aspects may be. Let's delve into why nurturing your emotional and psychological wellness can profoundly influence not just the length, but the richness of your life. From mastering stress management techniques to the priceless value of quality sleep and the transformative practices of mindfulness and meditation, this chapter will arm you with essential strategies to fortify the mind-body connection crucial for long-term vitality.

Stress Management Techniques

We all know life is full of stressors, from daily work pressures to personal challenges, and how we handle these stressors plays a critical role in our overall mental health. Effective stress management techniques are more than just a good-to-have; they are indispensable tools for achieving a longer, healthier, and happier life.

Let's dive into some tried-and-true methods that are not only powerful but also practical. If you've got a chaotic schedule, you might be skeptical about where to start. But guess what? Managing stress doesn't require you to overhaul your life; sometimes, it's the little changes that make the most significant impact.

Mindfulness Meditation

Mindfulness meditation is one of the most potent techniques for reducing stress. The idea is simple: focus on the present moment without judgment. Mindfulness teaches you to observe your thoughts and feelings without getting caught up in them. Studies have shown that even a few minutes of mindfulness meditation a day can lower cortisol levels, improve focus, and enhance emotional resilience.

Find a quiet corner, sit comfortably, and close your eyes. Focus on your breath—how it feels going in and out. When thoughts or distractions come up, gently guide your focus back to your breath. It sounds elementary, but its benefits are profound. The more you practice, the better you get at maintaining this awareness, even during stressful situations.

Physical Activity

We often hear about the physical benefits of exercise, but its mental health benefits are equally compelling. Physical activity triggers the release of endorphins, the brain's natural stress relievers. Whether it's a brisk walk, a session at the gym, or some yoga in your living room, moving your body can help clear your mind.

Ever notice how a workout can shift your mood from anxious to calm? That's not just in your head—it's biology at work. Consistent exercise not only mitigates stress but also helps improve sleep, another critical factor in managing stress levels.

Journaling

Another effective method to manage stress is journaling. Writing down your thoughts and feelings can be incredibly cathartic. It allows you to process what's happening in your life, helping to make sense of chaotic or troubling events. Journaling can serve as a mental dump, where you unload stress and gain perspective on your experiences.

You don't need to write novels—just a few sentences about what's on your mind will do. Over time, you'll see patterns and triggers that you might not have otherwise noticed, offering insights into how to better manage your reactions to stress.

Breathing Exercises

Specific breathing techniques can instantly calm your nervous system. Consider the 4-7-8 technique: inhale through your nose for four seconds, hold your breath for seven seconds, and then exhale through your mouth for eight seconds. This method activates your parasympathetic nervous system, encouraging a state of relaxation.

You can practice these exercises anywhere—at your desk, in your car, or even while waiting for your coffee. They're portable stress busters that can make a real difference in how you manage daily stressors.

Time Management

Effective time management is an often-overlooked aspect of stress management. When you're constantly racing against the clock, stress becomes a permanent fixture in your life. Create a schedule that allows for work, relaxation, and social time. Prioritize tasks, delegate responsibilities, and don't be afraid to say no. Setting boundaries protects your mental peace.

Try using tools like planners, to-do lists, or digital apps to streamline your tasks. Having a well-structured day reduces the last-minute rush and the anxiety that comes with it.

Social Connections

Humans are inherently social beings, and strong social connections are vital for our mental health. Whether it's a family gathering, a friendly chat, or even a call to someone who gets you, these connections can be a tremendous stress buffer. It's not just about having people around; it's about feeling supported and understood.

Make it a point to connect with loved ones regularly. It doesn't have to be grandiose or time-consuming. Sometimes, a simple "How are you?" can go a long way in lifting spirits and easing stress.

Relaxation Techniques

We often underestimate the value of doing nothing. Engaging in relaxation techniques such as progressive muscle relaxation, guided imagery, or listening to calming music can be incredibly beneficial. These methods decrease heart rate, relieve tension, and improve mood.

Reframe Your Thoughts

Cognitive reframing involves changing the way you look at a situation to alter your emotional response to it. Instead of thinking, "I can't handle this," consider thinking, "I will do my best, and that's enough." By reframing negative or stressful thoughts, you reduce the stress they cause.

It's a mental exercise but also a life-changer. Training your mind to focus on positive aspects or to see challenges as opportunities rather than threats makes a significant difference.

Healthy Lifestyle Choices

Opt for a balanced diet, stay hydrated, and ensure you get quality sleep. These fundamental health practices affect your body's ability to cope with stress. Poor lifestyle choices can aggravate stressors and decrease your resilience.

Maintaining physical health can complement your stress management efforts. Healthy body, healthy mind, as they say.

Seek Professional Help

Sometimes stress can be overwhelming, and there's no shame in seeking professional help. Therapists, counselors, and life coaches can offer personalized strategies to manage stress. Just having an outsider's perspective can offer new insights and solutions you hadn't considered.

Remember, asking for help is a strength, not a weakness. Professional guidance can provide you with tailored strategies to suit your unique challenges and lifestyle.

Addressing stress isn't about eliminating it entirely—after all, life will always have its ups and downs. It's about managing it effectively, so it doesn't take over your life. From mindfulness to movement, from breathing exercises to better time management, these techniques can empower you to lead a balanced, harmonious life.

Incorporate these strategies into your daily routine, and you'll find that not only your mental health improves, but your overall quality of life does as well. Let's reclaim our peace, one mindful breath at a time.

The Importance of Sleep

Ah, sleep. It's something we sometimes sacrifice in our fast-paced lives, but the truth is, sleep is one of the most powerful tools we have for maintaining mental health. When you're getting enough high-quality shut-eye, your brain functions at its best, which means better mood regulation, increased cognitive function, and a greater ability to manage stress. Think of sleep as your body's nightly reset button. It's during those restful hours that your brain processes emotions and memories, making it essential not just for your body, but also for a rock-solid mind. Prioritizing sleep isn't just about feeling more rested;

it's about giving your brain the chance to heal and rejuvenate. So, if you're aiming for a longer, happier life, don't skimp on those zzz's. Trust me, your future self will thank you.

Sleep Hygiene Tips may sound like a fancy term, but it's really all about creating habits that foster high-quality sleep. High-quality sleep isn't a luxury—it's an absolute necessity for a long and healthy life. You might think sleep just helps you feel refreshed, but it's so much more than that. It's deeply tied to your mental health, immune system, and longevity.

Let's start with your sleep environment. Creating a sanctuary for sleep means paying attention to your bedroom's setup. Your room should be cool, dark, and quiet. Think of it as a cave—this is where your body feels most at ease. An optimal room temperature is around 60-67°F (15-19°C). If the light sneaks in, blackout curtains can be your best friends. And don't overlook the power of white noise machines or earplugs to block out intrusive sounds.

Another important factor is your mattress and pillows. You spend a third of your life sleeping, so investing in comfortable bedding isn't just about luxury; it's a health investment. A supportive mattress can alleviate tension in your body, promoting relaxation. Similarly, pillows that support your neck properly can prevent stiffness and pain.

Now, let's dive into the nitty-gritty details of pre-sleep habits. Your body thrives on routine. Going to bed and waking up at the same time every day helps regulate your circadian rhythm, the internal clock responsible for making you feel sleepy or alert. Consistency reinforces your body's natural sleep-wake cycle.

Pay close attention to what you consume. Avoid heavy meals, caffeine, and alcohol before bedtime. While alcohol might make you feel drowsy initially, it can disrupt your sleep later in the night.

Caffeine, on the other hand, can linger in your system for hours, reducing your ability to fall asleep and stay asleep.

Engage in winding-down activities. Reading a book, doing some gentle stretches, or listening to soothing music can help transition your mind and body into a state of relaxation. Avoid screens at least an hour before bed. Devices emit blue light that tricks your brain into thinking it's still daytime, suppressing melatonin production, the hormone responsible for sleepiness.

Speaking of melatonin, consider creating a soothing bedtime routine that signals to your brain it's time to sleep. You could take a warm bath, which initially raises your body temperature and then causes it to drop, mimicking the natural drop in body temperature that signals sleep. Practicing mindfulness or deep breathing exercises can also be highly effective. These techniques help to calm your mind and reduce stress, making it easier to drift off.

Why stop at relaxation techniques? Embrace the healing power of scents. Aromatherapy with essential oils like lavender, chamomile, or sandalwood can make your sleep environment even more inviting. Just a few drops on your pillow or in a diffuser can make a world of difference in creating a peaceful atmosphere.

Your relationship with sleep should also extend into the daytime. Expose yourself to natural light during the day, especially morning sunlight. Natural light helps calibrate your internal clock. Engaging in physical activity during the day can also help you fall asleep more easily at night. However, try to finish vigorous exercises at least a few hours before bed.

What about naps? While napping can be beneficial, it's essential to approach it wisely. Short naps of 20-30 minutes can be rejuvenating, but longer naps can interfere with your nighttime sleep. If you find you need long naps, it could be a sign you're not getting enough quality sleep at night.

It's also worth monitoring your mental health. Worry and anxiety can sabotage your efforts to get a good night's sleep. Journaling before bed can help you process and calm racing thoughts. Writing down what's on your mind gets it out of your head, making it easier to unwind.

Let's not overlook the role of Tech in our sleep hygiene. We live in a digital world, and while there are downsides, technology can also help improve sleep. Apps that track sleep patterns, use white noise, or guide you through relaxation exercises can be valuable tools. Just make sure to use them wisely and not right before bedtime.

Your bed should be associated with sleep and relaxation. Avoid working, eating, or watching TV in bed. This trains your brain to associate your bed exclusively with rest, making it easier to fall asleep and stay asleep. The more you reinforce this association, the more you'll condition yourself for restful slumber.

Lastly, if you wake up in the middle of the night and can't fall back asleep within 20 minutes, get out of bed and do something quietly relaxing. Read a book, meditate, or listen to calming music. Avoid screens and bright lights. When you start feeling sleepy, go back to bed. This technique prevents you from associating your bed with wakefulness.

Your journey to optimal health and longevity is incomplete without prioritizing sleep. The habits you cultivate around sleep hygiene will ripple across every facet of your well-being. As you fine-tune these practices, you'll likely notice more than just better sleep: you'll find a renewed sense of energy, mental clarity, and emotional balance. So, take these sleep hygiene tips to heart—your future self will thank you.

Mindfulness and Meditation

Mental health is an integral component of overall wellness, especially when it comes to extending one's lifespan and improving quality of life. Among the myriad tools available for achieving optimal mental health, mindfulness and meditation stand out as two of the most powerful. They offer a holistic approach to mental well-being, addressing everything from stress and anxiety to sleep and emotional balance. These practices are not just for monks and yogis; they are accessible to everyone, regardless of age, background, or lifestyle.

Mindfulness, at its core, is about being fully present in the moment. It means paying attention to your thoughts, feelings, and surroundings without judgment. Sounds simple, right? Yet in a world filled with constant distractions, being truly mindful can be challenging. Smartphones, social media, and the relentless pace of modern life make it easy to drift through your days on autopilot. But here's the good news: anyone can cultivate mindfulness with practice and intention.

Meditation, while closely related to mindfulness, is a more structured practice aimed at achieving heightened awareness and mental clarity. There are numerous types of meditation - from guided meditations and mantra chanting to transcendental meditation and loving-kindness practices. Whether you prefer sitting quietly and focusing on your breath or using a meditation app, the key is consistency. Even just a few minutes a day can make a world of difference.

Imagine starting your day with a brief period of meditation. As you sit quietly, focusing on your breath, you begin to notice the thoughts that float through your mind. Rather than getting tangled up in them, you simply acknowledge them and let them go. This simple practice can set the tone for a calmer, more focused day. Studies have shown that meditation can reduce stress, enhance concentration, and even improve immune function.

Incorporating mindfulness into your daily routine doesn't require hours of sitting cross-legged on a cushion. It can be as simple as being present during mundane activities. For example, while brushing your teeth, pay attention to the sensation of the bristles against your gums, the taste of the toothpaste, and the sound of the running water. By consistently bringing your mind back to the present moment, you train yourself to be more mindful in all aspects of life.

The benefits of mindfulness and meditation extend far beyond stress reduction. They have been linked to improved emotional regulation, better sleep, and increased resilience. By becoming more aware of your thoughts and feelings, you can gain greater control over your reactions to life's challenges. This can lead to healthier relationships, improved decision-making, and a more positive outlook on life.

Mindfulness and meditation also play a crucial role in mitigating the effects of aging on the brain. Research has shown that regular practice can lead to increased gray matter in regions of the brain associated with memory, learning, and emotional regulation. Just as physical exercise strengthens the body, mental exercises like meditation strengthen the mind. This can be particularly beneficial as we age, helping to maintain cognitive function and emotional well-being.

But perhaps the most transformative aspect of mindfulness and meditation is the shift in perspective they offer. By fostering a deeper connection to the present moment, you begin to appreciate the richness of life's experiences more fully. This sense of presence can enhance your overall well-being and bring a profound sense of peace and contentment.

In our quest for longevity, it's easy to focus on the physical aspects of health - diet, exercise, sleep. But mental health is equally important. By incorporating mindfulness and meditation into your routine, you create a foundation for a balanced, healthy life. You'll find that you're not just living longer, but living better.

To start, find a quiet space where you won't be disturbed. Sit comfortably, close your eyes, and take a few deep breaths. Focus on the sensation of the breath entering and leaving your body. When your mind wanders, gently bring it back to the breath. If you prefer guided instruction, there are countless resources available, from apps to online courses, that can help you get started.

As you become more comfortable with the practice, you may choose to explore different types of meditation. Guided meditations, where an instructor leads you through the process, can be especially helpful for beginners. Body scan meditations focus on bringing awareness to different parts of the body, promoting relaxation and stress relief. Loving-kindness meditations cultivate feelings of compassion and empathy, enhancing emotional well-being.

The key to successful mindfulness and meditation practice is consistency. Like any new habit, it takes time to see the benefits. But with regular practice, you'll likely find that you feel calmer, more focused, and more in tune with yourself. Remember, there is no right or wrong way to meditate. The goal is not to achieve a perfect state of mind but to cultivate a sense of awareness and presence.

For those days when formal meditation feels daunting, try incorporating mindfulness into your daily activities. While eating, savor each bite, noticing the flavors, textures, and aromas of your food. During a walk, pay attention to the sights, sounds, and sensations around you. These moments of mindful awareness can add up, contributing to a greater sense of peace and well-being.

It can also be helpful to establish a routine that supports your practice. Perhaps you start your day with a few minutes of meditation, take a mindful walk during lunch, and wind down in the evening with a body scan meditation. Over time, these practices will become second nature, seamlessly integrating into your daily life.

If you're new to mindfulness and meditation, it can be helpful to start with short sessions and gradually increase the duration as you become more comfortable. Even a few minutes a day can have a significant impact on your mental health over time. Be patient with yourself, and remember that the journey is just as important as the destination.

Community can also play a significant role in supporting your mindfulness and meditation practice. Consider joining a meditation group or taking a class to connect with others who share your interest. Online communities and forums can also provide valuable support and resources. Sharing your experiences and challenges with others can deepen your understanding and commitment to the practice.

In conclusion, incorporating mindfulness and meditation into your life can profoundly impact your mental health and overall well-being. These practices offer a simple but powerful way to cultivate presence, reduce stress, and enhance your quality of life. As you continue your journey towards optimal health and longevity, remember that the mind is just as important as the body. By nurturing both, you create the foundation for a balanced, fulfilling life.

Chapter 5:
The Social Connection

Imagine a web that connects you to every person you care about and every social interaction you've ever had; this web is more than mere threads—it's a lifeline to longevity. What you might not realize is that social connections can be as vital to your health as any diet or exercise routine. Studies consistently show that strong social ties can boost your immune system, lower stress levels, and even increase your life expectancy. Whether hanging out with friends, spending quality time with family, or simply engaging in community activities, these interactions nourish not just your soul but your body too. It's incredible how sharing a laugh or lending an ear can create invisible yet powerful bonds that enhance your well-being. So while it's essential to eat right and stay active, don't underestimate the power of a good conversation or a heartfelt hug; they're the social vitamins that can make a world of difference.

Building a Support Network

Navigating life's complexities becomes substantially easier when you have a strong support network. No man is an island, as the saying goes, and this holds especially true when it comes to enhancing your health and longevity. A support network isn't just about having people to lean on during tough times; it's about cultivating a community that uplifts you, shares your values, and pushes you to be better every day.

First and foremost, let's recognize the importance of family. Family ties are often the bedrock of our social networks. They provide a level of unconditional love and understanding that's hard to find elsewhere. It's valuable to nurture these relationships, even when life's demands make it challenging. Simple gestures, such as weekly calls or occasional family gatherings, can make a world of difference in strengthening these bonds.

On the other hand, not everyone has a supportive family, and that's perfectly okay. Friends can be just as significant, if not more so, in building your support network. Unlike family, you get to choose your friends, and they often reflect your values and interests more closely. So, make the effort to surround yourself with people who inspire, motivate, and challenge you in positive ways. They say you are the average of the five people you spend the most time with—make those five count.

Creating and maintaining friendships often requires effort and time. In today's fast-paced life, it can be hard to find the time, but it's worth it. Go out for coffee, join a book club, or even start a hobby group. These activities not only help build friendships but also keep your mind engaged and active.

It's crucial to engage in activities where you're likely to meet like-minded people. Community centers, fitness classes, and volunteering opportunities provide fertile ground for relationships to blossom. Imagine the synergy created by people coming together with shared goals—be it enhancing their mental health, engaging in a philanthropic cause, or simply leading a healthier lifestyle.

Consider the power of mentorship, both being a mentor and having one. Mentorship can provide a pathway to deeper connections, knowledge, and growth. A mentor can offer guidance, share life experiences, and provide a wealth of knowledge that only years of living can offer. Conversely, mentoring someone else allows you to impart your wisdom, keeping you engaged and connected to the younger generation.

Work or career-based networks also offer robust possibilities for support. Professional associations and industry conferences provide excellent forums for meeting individuals who share your professional interests. These connections can be both professionally enriching and personally fulfilling.

Technology, too, offers endless possibilities. While social media can sometimes feel isolating or superficial, when used wisely, it can be a powerful tool to build and maintain your support network. Groups on platforms like Facebook, LinkedIn, and even specialized forums for various interests can keep you connected with people who share your passions.

However, virtual connections shouldn't replace face-to-face interactions. The nuances of body language, the subtleties of a smile, and the warmth of a hug can't be replicated online. So make it a point to cultivate your virtual relationships into real-world connections whenever possible.

Your support network should also include healthcare professionals. Regular check-ins with doctors, therapists, and wellness coaches can offer you professional support and guidance. Don't underestimate the value of professional advice when it comes to maintaining your health and well-being.

Pets can be a surprisingly significant part of your support network. Anyone who has ever owned a pet knows the joy and companionship they bring. Research has shown that pets can help reduce stress, lower blood pressure, and even improve overall mental health. They offer non-judgmental companionship and help us feel less lonely.

Don't forget the power of support groups, particularly if you're facing specific challenges or conditions. These groups provide an avenue to share experiences, gain emotional support, and learn coping strategies from others who are facing similar issues.

Being part of a support network doesn't mean only receiving help. It's also about reciprocating and providing support to others. This reciprocity builds a more resilient and connected community, fostering an environment where everyone thrives.

It's also worth mentioning the importance of setting boundaries. While it's essential to have a support network, it's equally important to ensure that this network remains healthy and constructive. Toxic relationships can undermine your well-being, so it's crucial to recognize and address them appropriately.

Don't be afraid to ask for help or express your needs. Often, people are more than willing to help but don't know what you need until you communicate it. Clear communication can go a long way in strengthening your relationships and ensuring that your support network functions effectively.

In conclusion, building a support network is not a task to be taken lightly. It requires effort, intentionality, and, most importantly, a genuine desire to connect. But the rewards—enhanced well-being, a sense of belonging, and the comfort of knowing you're not alone—make it all worthwhile. The journey to optimal health and longevity is not meant to be walked alone, and with a strong support network, you'll find the journey much more enriching and joyful.

The Impact of Loneliness

We live in an era where the paradox of connection is starkly evident. Even with the advent of social media and digital communication, cases of loneliness have skyrocketed to unprecedented levels. It's essential to recognize that loneliness isn't just a fleeting feeling—it's a powerful, chronic stressor with profound effects on our health and longevity.

Loneliness can be as lethal as smoking 15 cigarettes a day. Studies have shown that social isolation can increase the risk of premature death by 50%. The physiological impacts are tangible, affecting everything from our immune system to our cardiovascular health. It's not just an emotional struggle; it's a health crisis.

Our biology craves connection. Humans are inherently social beings. When isolated, our bodies react as if they're under attack. Cortisol, the stress hormone, spikes, leading to inflammation and a host of other health issues. Chronic loneliness has been linked to conditions such as hypertension, heart disease, and even neurodegenerative diseases like Alzheimer's.

But why does loneliness affect us so deeply? Consider this: our ancestors relied on their tribes for survival. Social bonds meant better protection, resources, and chances of surviving dangers. This ingrained need for connection hasn't changed, even though our living circumstances have. When we feel lonely, it's as if our bodies still think we're in danger of exclusion from our tribe.

Psychologically, the impact of loneliness is profound. It often feeds into cycles of negative thinking, self-doubt, and depression. This mental state can be just as damaging as physical illness. When someone feels isolated, their cognitive function can decline, and their ability to think clearly and make decisions may be impaired. It's not an overstatement to say that loneliness can cloud the mind.

Loneliness doesn't discriminate. It affects people of all ages and backgrounds. Adolescents can feel it in the hyper-connected world of social media. Adults might experience it while juggling responsibilities without meaningful support. Seniors often face it as they retire and lose lifelong relationships. And the COVID-19 pandemic has only exacerbated these feelings of isolation for many.

Ironically, loneliness can make it harder to reach out. Once someone feels isolated, they might find it challenging to initiate social interactions, fearing rejection or judgment. This creates a vicious cycle that can be tough to break. Recognizing the signs of loneliness in ourselves and others is the first step in combating it.

While the effects of loneliness are formidable, the solutions can be surprisingly simple yet powerful. Building and nurturing a support network is crucial. Sometimes, it's the little things—a meaningful conversation, a smile, or a shared activity—that can bridge the gap. Cultivating meaningful relationships should be a priority, much like maintaining a healthy diet or regular exercise.

Community involvement can be a game-changer. Volunteering, joining clubs, or participating in group activities can provide a sense of belonging. These activities not only offer social interaction but also bring a sense of purpose and fulfillment. The key is consistency and genuine engagement in these relationships and activities.

The power of pets shouldn't be underestimated, either. For many, a pet can provide companionship and reduce feelings of loneliness. Studies have shown that pet owners often have lower blood pressure and reduced levels of stress. The simple act of caring for another living being can bring tremendous emotional rewards.

Technology, when used mindfully, can also be a tool against loneliness. Video calls, online communities, and social media can help maintain connections, especially when in-person meetings are challenging. However, it's crucial to balance digital interactions with face-to-face time to nurture deeper, more meaningful relationships.

In professional settings, fostering a sense of community can alleviate workplace loneliness. Businesses can play a significant role by encouraging team-building activities and creating an inclusive work environment. When employees feel connected to their colleagues, job satisfaction and productivity often improve.

The role of mental health support in addressing loneliness cannot be overstated. Therapists and counselors can provide invaluable help, offering strategies to build social skills and cope with feelings of isolation. For many, professional guidance can be the catalyst for significant positive change.

In today's fast-paced world, the mantra of 'stop and smell the roses' holds more weight than ever. Being present and appreciative of the relationships we do have can make a massive difference. Gratitude practices, such as keeping a journal of positive interactions, can shift our mindset from what we lack to what we cherish.

Building a support network doesn't happen overnight; it requires effort, openness, and time. The rewards, however, are worth every bit of the investment. The more connected we feel, the healthier and happier we become. And this is a gift that keeps on giving, for ourselves and for the community around us.

In conclusion, loneliness is more than just a passing emotion. It's a serious health risk that can significantly affect one's quality of life and longevity. Yet, with awareness and proactive steps, it is a challenge that can be overcome. By fostering genuine connections, engaging in community activities, and seeking professional help when needed, we can conquer loneliness and unlock a healthier, longer, and more fulfilling life.

Chapter 6:
Environmental Factors

Imagine your home as a sanctuary, a place where every element is geared toward nourishing your well-being and extending your lifespan. The quality of the air you breathe, the water you drink, and the materials surrounding you can have profound effects on your health. Simple choices like opting for organic cleaning products, reducing plastic usage, and incorporating more natural light can create a harmonious living environment, free from harmful toxins. It's essential to consider not just what you put in your body, but also what you immerse your body in daily. By making mindful adjustments to your surroundings, you're not just adding years to your life, but life to your years. Trust that these small yet impactful changes can significantly boost your overall health, making your home a true haven for longevity.

Creating a Healthy Home Environment

Your home should be a sanctuary, a space where you can recharge and foster well-being. Crafting a healthy home environment isn't just about aesthetics; it's about creating a nurturing space that promotes longevity and quality of life. Think of your home as an extension of your body and mind, a place filled with the energies that either uplift or drain you.

Start with air quality. Many people underestimate the impact of clean air on their health. Indoor air pollutants, such as dust, mold, and volatile organic compounds (VOCs) from household products, can significantly affect your respiratory health. An air purifier can work wonders. It's like adding a breath of fresh air to your daily life, literally. Don't forget about natural ventilation either. Opening windows and allowing fresh air to circulate can reduce the concentration of indoor pollutants.

Water quality should also be on your radar. The human body is composed predominantly of water, so the quality of the water you consume matters a great deal. Investing in a good water filter can remove harmful contaminants and make a big difference to your overall health. Not all filters are created equal, so do your research to choose one that best suits your needs.

Paints, furniture, and cleaning products often harbor hidden toxins. Opt for low-VOC or VOC-free products where possible. This simple switch can minimize your exposure to harmful chemicals, creating a safer living space. Filling your home with plants can also help purify the air. Varieties like spider plants, snake plants, and pothos are particularly effective at removing toxins.

Lighting sets the mood of your home and can even impact your circadian rhythms, which are essential for good sleep. Natural light is best, so keep blinds and curtains open during the day. For artificial lighting, use LED bulbs that mimic daylight to help maintain your body's natural rhythms. At night, switch to softer, warmer lights to signal to your body that it's time to wind down.

When it comes to furnishings, comfort is paramount. Your home should be a place where you can relax and recover from the stresses of the day. A supportive mattress and ergonomic furniture can alleviate physical discomfort and contribute to better rest and productivity. Aim for a clutter-free space. Clutter isn't just an eyesore; it can also create mental stress. Less clutter fosters a more tranquil mind.

Your kitchen plays a central role in your health journey, too. Keep it organized and well-stocked with healthy, whole foods. Make your kitchen a place where nutritious meals can easily come together, making it more likely that you'll stick to your dietary goals. Keeping unhealthy snacks out of sight can reduce temptation and make it easier to choose wholesome options.

Don't forget about electronics. Minimize exposure to electromagnetic fields (EMFs) by keeping electronic devices out of the bedroom, especially where you sleep. Blue light emitted from screens can disrupt your sleep patterns, so limiting screen time before bed is crucial. Use blue-light filters on your devices if necessary.

The sense of smell can also significantly impact your well-being. Essential oils like lavender, eucalyptus, and peppermint can lift your mood and promote relaxation. Using a diffuser can distribute these healing scents throughout your home, creating an inviting and serene atmosphere.

Tending to your emotional and mental health is just as crucial. Create spaces for relaxation, meditation, or hobbies that bring joy. Whether it's a cozy reading nook or a corner for meditation, having designated areas for these activities can enrich your daily life. A space that reflects your interests and passions can be an ongoing source of inspiration and happiness.

Finally, relationships are just as much a part of your home environment as the physical space itself. Establish a home where relationships can flourish. Make room for shared activities and dining areas where family and friends can come together. A supportive environment filled with love and laughter will positively influence your emotional well-being.

Creating a healthy home environment involves a myriad of small choices that add up to a significant impact on your health and longevity. By taking these steps, you are not just creating a physical space, but nurturing a sanctuary that supports every aspect of your well-being. Let's transform our homes into spaces that truly enhance the quality of our lives. This isn't just about living longer—it's about living better.

Reducing Exposure to Toxins

We live in a world filled with invisible enemies. They're not the stuff of blockbuster movies but everyday toxins that seep into our lives, often unnoticed. It's crucial to guard ourselves against these invaders to ensure a longer, healthier life. You might be thinking, how big of a deal can a little exposure be? Well, let's dive in and see.

First off, why should we even care about reducing our exposure to toxins? These substances can disrupt our body's delicate balance, leading to a host of health issues — from minor irritations to serious diseases like cancer. The good news is, with a little awareness and some strategic changes, you can significantly decrease your exposure.

One of the first places to start is with the air you breathe. Indoor air can be up to five times more polluted than outdoor air. That's a lot of unwanted particles making their way into your lungs. Simple changes, like using an air purifier, keeping windows open for ventilation, and opting for non-toxic household cleaners, can make a world of difference. And let's not forget those sneaky off-gassing products like new furniture and carpets. Give them some time to air out before bringing them inside.

Let's take a closer look at household cleaning products. Have you ever looked at the ingredient list on a bottle of cleaner? Terms like "ammonia," "chlorine," and "phthalates" might appear. These harsh chemicals can linger in the air and on surfaces long after you've finished cleaning. Switching to natural cleaners made from ingredients like vinegar, baking soda, and essential oils can reduce your home's toxic load significantly. Plus, they often smell better too!

Next up, personal care products. The lotions, shampoos, and cosmetics we use daily can be a source of toxic exposure. Our skin is incredibly absorbent, meaning harmful chemicals in these products can enter our bloodstream pretty quickly. Look out for products free from parabens, sulfates, and synthetic fragrances. Brands are increasingly offering cleaner, greener options that still deliver on performance.

Food and water are another major exposure route for toxins. Pesticides, herbicides, and heavy metals can infiltrate our food supply. Opting for organic produce whenever possible can reduce your intake of these harmful chemicals. If going fully organic is out of budget, prioritize purchasing organic for the "dirty dozen" – those fruits and veggies most likely to be contaminated with pesticides.

Water quality is also a biggie. Even though the U.S. has some of the safest drinking water in the world, contaminants like lead, chlorine, and even pharmaceutical residues can still sneak in. Investing in a good water filter for your tap, and maybe even a shower filter, is a smart move. You'll be surprised at how much better the water tastes too!

Let's not forget the impact of plastics. From the containers we store our food in to the bottles we drink from, plastics can leach harmful chemicals like BPA and phthalates. These substances are endocrine disruptors, which can wreak havoc on our hormonal systems. Switching to glass or stainless steel containers, especially for hot food and drinks, is a step in the right direction.

Now, electronics might not be the first thing that comes to mind when thinking about toxins, but they can be a stealthy source of exposure. The screens, batteries, and circuit boards contain various heavy metals and flame retardants. Make sure to recycle electronics properly to prevent these hazardous materials from ending up in landfills, where they can contaminate soil and water supplies.

Lastly, let's talk about one often-overlooked area: the workplace. Depending on your job, you might be exposed to various chemicals and pollutants. Advocating for a safer work environment is critical. This might involve using protective gear, ensuring proper ventilation, and following best practices for handling hazardous materials.

Reducing your exposure to toxins doesn't mean you have to live in a bubble. It's about making informed choices and small adjustments that add up over time. Think of it as investing in your future self. Each toxin you avoid is a step towards a healthier, longer life, brimming with energy and vitality.

Take a moment to reflect on your current lifestyle. Where can you make changes? Is it in the products you use, the air you breathe, or the food you eat? Start with one area and make gradual improvements. You'd be surprised how these small changes can create a ripple effect, positively impacting not just your health, but also the health of those around you.

We might not be able to eliminate every toxin from our life, but we can certainly tilt the scales in our favor. Be mindful of your choices, stay informed, and keep striving for a life that's not just long, but full of health and joy. Here's to a cleaner, toxin-free world!

Chapter 7:
Ancient Wisdom Meets
Modern Science

Imagine a world where centuries-old healing traditions join forces with today's cutting-edge scientific breakthroughs to create a truly holistic approach to health. In this chapter, we dive into the rich tapestry of ancient practices like Ayurveda, Traditional Chinese Medicine, and indigenous healing, showing how these time-tested techniques can harmonize with modern science to enhance our well-being. We explore how these practices, often dismissed as mere folklore, are now being validated by contemporary research, providing new avenues for preventing disease and increasing longevity. With an open mind and a spirit of curiosity, you'll discover how blending ancient wisdom with modern methodologies can offer powerful tools for optimizing your health and vitality.

Traditional Medicine Practices

It's incredible to see how modern science is beginning to validate what many ancient cultures have known for centuries—that traditional medicine practices can play a significant role in promoting health and longevity. The fusion of ancient wisdom with cutting-edge research can provide us with unique insights into holistic wellness. Imagine combining centuries-old herbal remedies with modern nutritional science; it's like having the best of both worlds at your fingertips.

One of the cornerstones of traditional medicine practices is Ayurveda, a system that originated in India more than 3,000 years ago. Ayurveda focuses on balancing the body's three doshas—Vata, Pitta, and Kapha—to ensure optimal health. This holistic approach involves not just medicinal herbs but also diet, exercise, and spiritual well-being. Incorporating Ayurvedic principles into your daily life doesn't have to be complex. Simple practices like drinking warm water in the morning or including turmeric in your diet can make a world of difference.

Traditional Chinese Medicine (TCM) is another wellspring of ancient wisdom that complements modern scientific findings. Acupuncture, one of TCM's most well-known practices, has been shown to improve various ailments, from chronic pain to digestive disorders. The philosophy here is all about the flow of Qi, the vital life force that traverses your body through meridians. When you harmonize your Qi, you're essentially promoting balance and removing blockages that could lead to illness. Isn't it fascinating how tiny needles can wield such profound benefits?

Herbal medicine also holds a treasure trove of ancient remedies that have stood the test of time. Herbs like ginseng, ginkgo biloba, and ashwagandha have been used for centuries to enhance vitality and longevity. Modern research is now catching up, with numerous studies confirming their benefits. For instance, ginseng has been shown to improve cognitive function, while ashwagandha is renowned for its stress-relieving properties. Next time you're considering a supplement, why not look to these time-honored herbs?

Native American medicine also provides extraordinary insights into holistic well-being. Rooted in a deep respect for nature, these practices often involve using plants to treat illnesses and promote health. Smudging, or burning sage to purify the air, is a practice that's gaining popularity today not just for its spiritual benefits but also for its potential antimicrobial properties. There's something grounding about reconnecting with nature through these age-old rituals.

African traditional medicine is another ocean of knowledge, often overlooked but incredibly potent. Herbal concoctions, spiritual healing, and the use of charms and rituals form the cornerstone of these practices. African healers have an extensive pharmacopeia of plants and herbs that are just starting to be explored by modern science. For example, the African sausage tree (Kigelia Africana) is used for its antimicrobial and anti-inflammatory properties. How amazing is it that answers to our health issues might be growing right in our backyards?

One can't discuss traditional medicine without mentioning the rich practices of Indigenous Australian healing. The use of bush medicine, derived from the native flora, is central to their approach. Plants like eucalyptus and tea tree have been used for their antiseptic qualities long before they became staples in modern natural remedies. Integrating these practices into your wellness routine can provide both physical and spiritual benefits.

Shamanic healing, found in various cultures around the world, incorporates elements of spirituality, ritual, and herbal medicine. Shamans often act as intermediaries between the human and spirit worlds, using drumming, chanting, and plant medicines to facilitate healing. While this might sound mystical, it's interesting to note that many shamanic practices also incorporate knowledge of the medicinal properties of plants, proving yet again that ancient wisdom is intricately tied to the natural world.

When you think about traditional medicine, it's clear that it embraces a holistic view of health. Instead of focusing solely on symptoms, these practices encourage balance between mind, body, and spirit. This is a lesson that modern medicine is only beginning to learn. Techniques like yoga and Tai Chi, which originated in ancient traditions, are now widely recognized for their benefits in promoting mental and physical health. Incorporating these practices can help you achieve a more balanced and fulfilling life.

However, it's important to approach traditional medicine practices with an informed perspective. While these methods offer immense benefits, they should complement, not replace, modern medical treatments. Collaborating with healthcare providers to integrate traditional practices ensures that you get the best of both worlds. Always consult a qualified practitioner before starting any new health regimen, especially if you have underlying health conditions.

The fusion of traditional and modern medicine is a burgeoning field teeming with possibilities. Imagine a world where your healthcare plan includes consultations with both a doctor and an acupuncturist, or where your prescription includes both pharmaceutical drugs and herbal remedies. This integrative approach can provide a more comprehensive and personalized pathway to health and longevity.

It's clear that traditional medicine practices offer a rich tapestry of knowledge and techniques that can significantly enhance our modern health practices. These methods remind us to listen to our bodies, respect the natural world, and strive for balance in all aspects of our lives. As you explore these ancient wisdoms, you're not just adopting practices; you're embracing a philosophy that values holistic well-being.

There's no denying that we've come a long way in understanding health and longevity, yet there's so much to learn from the time-tested traditions of our ancestors. Whether it's through herbal remedies, holistic practices, or spiritual rituals, traditional medicine provides a well-rounded approach to health that can enrich our lives in countless ways. So, as you delve deeper into your wellness journey, remember to keep an open mind and heart, and let the wisdom of the ages guide you.

And remember—the journey to optimal health is a mosaic. Each piece, whether it's a traditional practice or a modern breakthrough, adds to the beautiful, complex picture of a long and fulfilling life. This integration of ancient and contemporary knowledge doesn't just offer you remedies; it provides a roadmap for a life brimming with vitality and joy. So why not take a leaf from both the old and the new? You just might discover the best version of yourself waiting on the other side.

Integrating Holistic Approaches

Imagine a world where ancient healing traditions and cutting-edge science come together in a harmonious blend—we'd be taking a major leap towards optimizing our health and longevity. Integrating holistic approaches with modern scientific methods can provide a more comprehensive blueprint for well-being. But what does this integration look like in practice?

Let's start by understanding what we mean by holistic approaches. Holistic health isn't a single practice; it's a philosophy that takes into account the whole person—mind, body, and spirit. This includes nutrition, physical activity, emotional balance, and even spiritual fulfillment. Ancient cultures, from the Egyptians to the Traditional Chinese Medicine practitioners, have long appreciated this interconnectedness. Modern science now provides a framework for validating many of these age-old practices.

Consider acupuncture, an ancient Chinese practice that involves inserting thin needles at specific points on the body. Historically, it has been used to treat everything from chronic pain to digestive issues. Recent studies confirm its efficacy in pain management and stress reduction. By fusing ancient wisdom with modern clinical trials, we gain a broader understanding of its benefits and can more effectively incorporate it into our health regimens.

Yoga is another stellar example. Originating in ancient India, yoga combines physical postures, breathing exercises, and meditation. Modern research shows that yoga reduces stress, enhances brain function, and improves cardiovascular health. So, incorporating yoga into our daily routines isn't just about flexibility; it's also about fostering mental clarity and physical well-being. A commitment to yoga can serve as a bridge between ancient wisdom and modern wellness.

Similarly, Ayurvedic medicine, with its roots in India, emphasizes balance in bodily systems through diet, herbal treatments, and yogic breathing. Each person has a unique constitution or "dosha," and Ayurveda offers dietary and lifestyle recommendations tailored to these individual needs. When combined with modern genetic and metabolic testing, we can precisely tailor Ayurvedic principles to best serve each individual's health needs.

Even the act of mindful eating—a practice rooted in Buddhism—has found its way into contemporary nutritional science. Mindful eating encourages us to slow down and savor every bite, paying attention to hunger cues and emotional triggers for eating. Studies show this can lead to better digestion, more enjoyment of food, and even weight loss. By integrating mindful eating principles into modern dietary guidelines, we create eating habits that nourish both body and soul.

Of course, the integration of holistic approaches with modern science isn't without challenges. One barrier is the rigorous standard of proof required by modern scientific methods compared to the more experiential validation used in traditional practices. But we are finding ways to meet in the middle. For example, clinical trials on herbal supplements often corroborate their traditional uses, helping to bridge this gap.

Let's talk about the power of nature in healing. Forest bathing or "shinrin-yoku," a practice that originated in Japan, involves spending time in a forested area to boost mental health and immunity. Modern studies highlight the benefits of nature exposure, revealing reductions in cortisol levels, blood pressure, and improvements in mood. This ancient practice is a fantastic example of how traditional wisdom can offer profound health benefits that are just now being scientifically validated.

Breathwork also deserves mention. Ancient yogic pranayama techniques are now scientifically proven to reduce stress, improve lung capacity, and regulate emotional states. Techniques like diaphragmatic breathing or alternate nostril breathing can be incorporated into modern stress management programs with significant efficacy. These practices show the potential for integrating ancient breathwork with contemporary mental health strategies, offering accessible tools for emotional and physical well-being.

It's impossible to discuss holistic approaches without mentioning herbal medicine. Traditional cultures have long used plants and herbs like turmeric, ginger, and ginseng, for their health benefits. Current scientific research often supports these uses. Curcumin, the active compound in turmeric, is now recognized for its anti-inflammatory and antioxidant properties. We can integrate these findings into our diets through culinary practices or supplements, combining the wisdom of the past with contemporary nutritional science.

Meditation and mindfulness practices originating from the Buddhist tradition have also found a place in modern psychology. Techniques such as Mindfulness-Based Stress Reduction (MBSR) and Mindfulness-Based Cognitive Therapy (MBCT) demonstrate how ancient practices can evolve into clinically validated interventions. Integrating meditation into our daily lives can lower stress levels, improve emotional regulation, and enhance overall well-being.

Another significant area is energy healing, such as Reiki. While Western medicine initially viewed practices like Reiki with skepticism, growing evidence supports its role in stress reduction and emotional healing. Scientific studies measuring heart rate variability and biofield changes have begun to confirm what traditional practitioners have known for centuries. By adopting such approaches alongside conventional medical treatments, we open new avenues for healing.

The fusion of traditional nutritional practices with modern dietary science also exemplifies integration. Many cultures have inherent wisdom in their culinary traditions. For example, the Mediterranean diet, rich in olive oil, fish, and fresh vegetables, is now backed by modern research promoting cardiovascular health and longevity. By embracing these time-tested dietary patterns, we leverage both ancestral knowledge and current nutritional insights.

Holistic approaches aren't just about individual practices but also about the lifestyle philosophy they embody. In regions with high life expectancies, such as the Blue Zones, we observe common holistic elements: strong social bonds, plant-based diets, regular physical activity, and a sense of purpose. Modern research supports these components as critical for long-term health. By understanding and adopting these lifestyle traits, we can craft a modern life rich in ancient wisdom.

Integrating holistic approaches with modern science means adopting an open, yet discerning, mindset. We should be willing to explore and validate traditional methods through the lens of contemporary research while maintaining respect for the intrinsic value these practices offer. This balanced view enables us to curate a comprehensive wellness strategy that honors the legacy of ancient traditions while embracing the advancements of modern science.

Incorporating holistic approaches into our lives doesn't have to be daunting or dogmatic. Start small. Introduce a mindfulness practice, try a new herb, or spend a mindful moment in nature. Over time, these small steps can lead to profound shifts in your overall well-being.

By synergizing ancient wisdom with modern science, we don't just extend our lives; we enrich them. We create a tapestry of health practices that honor time-tested traditions and the spirit of innovation. This integrated approach equips us with a versatile toolkit for navigating modern life's complexities while staying grounded in timeless principles of wellness. Together, we can craft a life that's not only longer but fuller and more vibrant.

Chapter 8:
Personalized Medicine

Imagine a world where your healthcare isn't based on general guidelines but is tailored specifically for you. That's the promise of personalized medicine. This innovative approach leverages genetic testing and other advanced diagnostics to create individualized health strategies designed to meet your unique needs. It's like having a roadmap created just for you, guiding you to optimum health and longevity. By understanding your genetic makeup, lifestyle, and environmental factors, personalized medicine empowers you to make informed decisions, tailoring health protocols that work best for your body and mind. This isn't just about treating illness; it's about cultivating a proactive, preventative mindset for lifelong well-being. As you embark on your journey with personalized medicine, remember, you're not just a patient—you're a partner in your own health.

Genetic Testing and Its Implications

If personalized medicine is the future, then genetic testing is the rocket fuel that will get us there. Just imagine the possibilities – knowing your genetic makeup could inform everything from the best diet for your body to how you should manage stress or sleep. It's not science fiction; it's science fact. Genetic testing can provide an extraordinary level of insight into our biological blueprint, allowing us to tailor our health protocols down to the tiniest detail. This is where the journey from generic health advice to precision medicine begins.

Think about the last time you took advice from a friend who swore that cutting out carbs transformed their life, only for you to find it left you lethargic and hangry. Or perhaps you've tried a popular workout regime that left you more injured than energized. These discrepancies exist because we aren't one-size-fits-all. Genetic testing promises to change all that by providing data tailored specifically to you. This isn't just a "nice-to-have." For those looking to optimize their health and longevity, understanding their genes is essential.

Genetic testing can offer insights into a myriad of health aspects, from your propensity for certain diseases to how you metabolize different nutrients. Can you imagine knowing that you have a genetic predisposition to be lactose intolerant rather than just figuring it out through years of stomach aches and guesswork? These tests can tell you that and so much more.

As powerful as this technology is, it's important to approach it with the right mindset. A genetic test isn't a fortune teller; it's a roadmap. It won't tell you everything, but it can give you essential signs and directions. Yes, you might find out you have a higher risk for conditions like heart disease or diabetes, but knowing this information is half the battle. With the knowledge gained from these tests, you can take actionable steps to mitigate these risks.

Incorporating genetic testing into your health regime isn't just about understanding what could go wrong. It's also about unlocking potential. Are you more likely to benefit from certain types of exercise over others? Does your body respond particularly well to plant-based diets? Genetic testing can give you tailored recommendations that help maximize your health gains.

It's worth noting that genetic testing goes beyond just physical health. Our genes can provide insights into our mental health as well. Some individuals might be more prone to anxiety or depression due to their genetic makeup. Understanding this can lead to proactive mental health strategies tailored to these predispositions, helping build stronger emotional resilience.

The impact of genetic testing on personalized medicine is profound. For instance, pharmacogenomics is a field that studies how genes affect a person's response to drugs. Imagine no longer having to suffer through trial and error with medications. Your genetic data can guide doctors in prescribing medications that will be most effective for you, minimizing side effects and enhancing efficacy. This can be particularly significant for complex conditions like cancer or chronic pain, where finding the right treatment can make a substantial difference in quality of life.

However, with great power comes great responsibility. The data derived from genetic testing is sensitive. It's your biological fingerprint. While the benefits are enormous, it raises ethical questions about privacy and data security. You'll have to consider how and where your genetic data is stored and who has access to it. Many companies have robust privacy measures in place, but it's always wise to do your own research before diving in.

Then there's the psychological aspect of knowing your genetic risks. Not everyone is prepared to learn they have a higher likelihood of developing a life-altering condition. However, knowledge is power. The emotional burden can be managed with the right support systems in place, such as counseling or support groups. Transparency with healthcare providers and loved ones can also help navigate the complexities that this knowledge brings.

Taking this a step further, think about the potential for family planning. Genetic tests can inform prospective parents about the likelihood of passing on certain genetic conditions to their children. This is invaluable information for those who want to make informed decisions about their family's future health.

Far from being a static snapshot of your genetic makeup, the landscape of genetic testing is rapidly evolving. New discoveries and technologies are continually emerging, making it an ever-more precise tool. Companies are not just looking at individual genes anymore; they're analyzing entire genomic sequences, offering a more holistic view of your health predispositions.

Let's not forget the societal implications. Widespread genetic testing could lead to better population health strategies. Public health policies could be tailored based on genetic trends within specific communities, leading to more effective interventions and preventive measures. This isn't just about individual health; it's about the collective well-being of society.

In summary, genetic testing is a groundbreaking tool that can profoundly affect your approach to health and longevity. It's about more than just knowing your risks; it's about empowering you to make proactive, informed decisions. As part of a comprehensive approach to personalized medicine, your genetic profile becomes a valuable asset in your quest for a longer, healthier life.

As you navigate through this transformative journey of self-discovery and optimized health, remember that you are not alone. Lean on the support of healthcare professionals, loved ones, and the expansive community of individuals who are equally committed to leveraging genetic insights for a better life. Embrace the knowledge not as a predestined fate but as a map towards the healthiest version of you.

Your genes are the script, but you hold the pen. Write a story of vitality, longevity, and well-being, armed with the power of genetic insight and personalized medicine.

Tailoring Health Protocols

Personalized medicine shines in its ability to sculpt health protocols that fit you like a glove. Imagine walking into a room tailor-made for your needs—each piece of furniture arranged to suit your comfort, every light adjusted to enhance your mood. This analogy holds true for tailoring health protocols in the realm of personalized medicine. By leveraging modern technology and scientific advancements, we can craft bespoke health plans that align uniquely with your genetic makeup, lifestyle, and specific health conditions.

In today's world, a one-size-fits-all approach to healthcare just doesn't cut it. The beauty of personalized medicine is in its flexibility. It's about recognizing that no two individuals are the same, and thus, their health strategies shouldn't be indistinguishable. This individualized approach transforms medicine from a reactive practice into a proactive journey, empowering you to steer the course of your own well-being with the precision of a finely tuned instrument.

Tailoring health protocols often begins with a deep dive into genetic testing. Your DNA is your body's instruction manual, a treasure trove of information. By decoding these instructions, we can better understand your unique health risks and predispositions. Whether it's identifying a single nucleotide polymorphism that affects how you metabolize caffeine or discovering a genetic mutation that increases your risk for a particular disease, the insights gleaned are invaluable. Armed with this knowledge, you can make informed decisions about your diet, exercise, and even medication.

But genetic information is merely the tip of the iceberg. Tailoring health protocols also involves taking a holistic look at your lifestyle. Do you spend hours hunched over a computer, or are you constantly on the move? Are you a night owl who struggles with sleep, or an early bird who wakes up with the sun? These lifestyle factors are crucial in crafting a health strategy that works for you. For instance, if you're prone to stress and anxiety, your health plan might include mindfulness practices and stress management techniques like yoga or meditation.

Moreover, your environment plays a significant role. Personalized medicine takes into account the toxins you're exposed to in your home or workplace, the quality of the air you breathe, and even the impact of your social connections. By understanding these factors, we can recommend adjustments that minimize your exposure to harmful elements and bolster your overall health.

Let's not overlook the power of nutrition. Tailoring health protocols means customizing your diet to meet your body's specific needs and optimize your health. Are you lactose intolerant? Do you have a sensitivity to gluten, or perhaps a need for more omega-3 fatty acids? Personalized nutrition plans take these unique requirements into account. We know that what works wonders for one person may not be beneficial for another. It's about finding the foods that fuel your body best, keeping inflammation at bay, and ensuring you get the right balance of nutrients to support longevity.

While the intricacies of genetics and lifestyle are significant, another pillar of tailored health protocols is continuous monitoring and adjustment. Think of it as the fine-tuning of a musical instrument; the process is iterative and ongoing. Health metrics from wearable devices can provide real-time data on your heart rate, sleep patterns, and activity levels. By consistently tracking these markers, adjustments can be made on the fly. If you're not getting enough REM sleep, simple tweaks to your evening routine might be introduced to help you rest better.

Perhaps one of the most thrilling aspects of personalized medicine is its dynamic nature. It's not static; it evolves with you. As new research emerges and as we gather more data from your unique health journey, these protocols can be refined. It's about staying agile and adaptable, ensuring that your health strategy remains as effective tomorrow as it is today. This is the crux of longevity—constantly evolving to meet the changing demands of your body and environment.

Motivation and inspiration are central to the success of tailored health protocols. Imagine knowing that each action you take is a step closer to a longer, healthier life uniquely designed for you. This is peak empowerment. When you understand the 'why' and 'how' behind your health choices, you're more likely to stick with them. Tailored health protocols offer not just a plan, but a purpose. Each meal, each workout, each moment of rest is not random but part of a greater strategy aimed at optimal living.

Every element of your health protocol is interwoven with all others, creating a harmonious balance that supports your well-being. For instance, integrating stress management techniques like deep breathing or tai chi can enhance your cardiovascular health and improve sleep quality. In turn, better sleep can boost your immune system and regulate hormones, leading to a more robust response to illness and stress. It's a wonderfully interconnected web where each thread reinforces the other.

Tailoring health protocols also extends to medication and supplement use. Genetic information can guide the choice of medications that are most effective for you, minimizing adverse reactions and maximizing benefits. Personalized supplement plans can target deficiencies or enhance your body's natural healing processes. Imagine skipping the trial-and-error phase and going straight to what works, based on a deep understanding of your biochemistry.

Finally, knowledge is the bedrock of personalized medicine. This entire process hinges on learning and understanding your unique health landscape. Whether it's through regular health check-ups, genetic testing, or consultations with healthcare providers, the goal is to gather as much relevant information as possible. The more you know, the more power you have to shape your health journey.

In conclusion, tailoring health protocols is about crafting a life strategy that's as unique as your fingerprint. It's about harnessing the power of modern science and ancient wisdom to design a roadmap that leads to optimal health and longevity. With each personalized adjustment, you're taking steps not just to live longer, but to live better. It's more than a health plan; it's a life philosophy that celebrates your uniqueness and fuels your potential. So, embrace this personalized journey and unlock the extraordinary potential of a life lived fully and healthily.

Chapter 9:
Preventative Healthcare

We often hear that "an ounce of prevention is worth a pound of cure," but what does that truly mean for our quest for longevity? Preventative healthcare is all about taking proactive steps to ward off illnesses before they start, ensuring you're not just adding years to your life but life to your years. This means booking those regular check-ups, staying on top of early detection strategies, and maintaining a keen awareness of your body's signals. Picture yourself as both the captain and the navigator of your health journey, steering clear of potential hazards long before they come into view. It's about cultivating a lifestyle where wellness checks and preemptive measures become as routine as brushing your teeth. Trust me, investing in prevention isn't just wise; it's transformative. This proactive approach can empower you with the resilience and vitality you need to take on life's adventures with vigor and grace.

Regular Health Check-Ups

Imagine you have a car. You wouldn't drive it for years without getting it serviced, would you? Regular health check-ups are essentially the tune-ups and oil changes your body needs. They're your opportunity to catch issues before they become major problems, to tweak and optimize your health so you can run smoothly for as long as possible.

Think of regular check-ups as your health radar. They allow you to detect potential health threats early. The key is consistency. A single check-up won't provide you with a full picture, but regular, ongoing assessments will. Just like you wouldn't only take your car in when it's broken down, you shouldn't wait for symptoms to appear before seeing a doctor. Prevention is always better than cure, and that's what these regular visits are all about.

Your Lifelong Health Partnership

One of the most valuable aspects of regular health check-ups is the relationship you develop with your healthcare provider. This isn't just about a transactional visit a few times a year; it's about building a partnership aimed at optimizing your long-term health. Your doctor gets to know you, your lifestyle, and your personal and family medical history, enabling them to make more informed recommendations and decisions.

The beauty of this partnership is that it enables a more personalized approach to your healthcare. Rather than a one-size-fits-all solution, your healthcare provider can tailor their advice and treatments to fit your specific needs and circumstances. This collaboration transforms your check-ups from mere routine to a bespoke experience designed to elevate your health.

Stay Ahead of the Game

Many serious health conditions begin quietly and remain symptomless until they have already caused considerable damage. Regular health check-ups act as a preemptive strike against these silent threats. Conditions like high blood pressure, high cholesterol, and even early-stage cancers can be detected through routine screenings. Discovering these issues sooner means treatment can begin earlier, enhancing your chances of recovery and reducing the severity of potential complications.

For example, routine blood tests can flag anomalies in your biomarkers that might indicate an underlying issue. Your blood sugar levels, liver function, and kidney performance are just some of the things that can be monitored. Bone density scans can help identify early signs of osteoporosis. Each of these tests provides a snapshot of your physical state, adding to the complete picture of your health.

Empower Yourself with Knowledge

Information is power, and regular health check-ups empower you with knowledge about your body. These visits are opportunities to get professional insights into what's happening internally. Have you been feeling fatigued? Is your sleep quality declining? You've got your platform to discuss these issues and get professional advice. You walk away from each appointment with more understanding, more control, and more confidence in your health journey.

It's also a time when you can discuss preventative measures. Vaccinations, lifestyle modifications, and nutritional advice all come into play. Preventive care is a cornerstone of longevity, and every check-up is a stepping stone in optimizing your well-being.

Peace of Mind is Priceless

There's also an emotional and psychological component to regular health check-ups that can't be overlooked. Knowing you're actively monitoring your health provides peace of mind. It's comforting to know that you're doing everything you can to stay healthy for the long run. This proactive approach not only mitigates anxiety around health concerns but also encourages a more positive outlook on life.

Regular Check-Ups: What to Expect

So, what exactly should you expect during these routine check-ups? Typically, a comprehensive evaluation includes a review of your medical history, a physical examination, and various diagnostic tests based on your age, gender, and risk factors. You might have your weight, height, and body mass index (BMI) checked, along with blood pressure and heart rate measurements. Blood tests and urine tests can be part of the mix, providing insights into your organ function, glucose levels, and more.

Your doctor may also conduct specific screenings for cancers, osteoporosis, and other conditions based on your risk factors. Your lifestyle choices, such as diet, exercise, smoking, and alcohol consumption, will also be discussed. This is a chance to receive personalized recommendations that can make a significant difference in your long-term health. Through these conversations, you gain actionable insights that you can implement in your daily life.

The Future of Check-Ups: Advanced Diagnostics and Technology

With advancements in medical technology, regular check-ups are becoming even more efficient and insightful. Wearable devices that monitor your heart rate, sleep patterns, and physical activity levels are now more accessible and can provide valuable data during your appointments. Genetic testing is also playing an increasingly important role in preventative healthcare, offering a more detailed risk profile for various conditions.

A combination of traditional methods and modern technology can provide a comprehensive overview of your health. Imagine having a complete digital record of your health, which you and your doctor can access and update in real-time. This integration of technology into healthcare is shaping the future of regular health check-ups, making them more personalized and effective than ever before.

Taking the First Step

The idea of regular check-ups might be daunting for some, but it's essential to take that first step. Book an appointment and start the conversation about your health. View it as an investment. The time and effort you put into these appointments will pay dividends in terms of a healthier, longer life. Over time, these routine visits will become less of a chore and more of a welcomed ritual in your health journey.

The Synergy of Preventative Healthcare

Ultimately, regular health check-ups are one piece of the larger puzzle of preventative healthcare. They work in synergy with other practices like proper nutrition, regular exercise, mental health maintenance, and a fulfilling social life. All these elements combine to create a strong foundation for a long, healthy, and vibrant life.

Start today. Make that appointment. Take control of your health journey, and let every check-up be a milestone in your quest for longevity. By making regular check-ups a priority, you're not just reacting to life; you're shaping it.

Early Detection Strategies

Early detection strategies are transformative tools that can help stave off many serious health conditions before they become unmanageable. Imagine the impact of catching an illness at its most treatable stage. It's akin to tuning up your car before a long road trip—ensuring that it's running smoothly prevents breakdowns along the way. In healthcare, being proactive rather than reactive is like having a superpower. Early detection doesn't just promise a better outcome; it also offers peace of mind, allowing you to focus on living your best life without constant worry hanging over your head.

Prevention is the foundation of early detection strategies. Systems like regular health screenings, diagnostic tests, and monitoring your body's biomarkers are crucial. But these aren't just medical terms; they're life-saving checkpoints. Routine screenings for cholesterol, blood pressure, and blood sugar levels act as your first line of defense. They provide essential early warnings before conditions escalate into chronic diseases. It's like having a weather forecast that tells you to carry an umbrella—it's all about anticipating problems and being prepared.

You must also pay attention to cancer screenings. Mammograms, Pap smears, colonoscopies, and PSA tests are not elective. They are crucial in detecting abnormalities long before symptoms appear. Many forms of cancer are far easier to treat when caught early. Take heart in knowing that early detection significantly increases survival rates for numerous cancers. In these scenarios, knowledge is power—and it's the kind of power that can save your life.

Innovations in technology have ushered in a new era of early detection. We now have access to non-invasive tests and wearables that help monitor our health in real-time. Devices like smartwatches can track your heart rate, detect irregularities, and even assist in identifying sleep apnea. Genetic testing has also become more accessible and can provide insights into your predisposition to various diseases, enabling you to take preemptive action. Imagine having a personalized roadmap that helps you navigate potential health risks tailored specifically to your genetic makeup.

Consider also microbiome testing. The gut-brain connection is no longer a theory but a well-documented avenue for maintaining optimal health. Knowing the composition of your gut microbiome can help you tailor your diet and lifestyle to ward off issues like inflammation, depression, and even some autoimmune diseases. This early detection strategy isn't about invasive procedures but about understanding your body's ecosystem better and making informed decisions based on that knowledge.

Let's talk about mental health, which too often goes unnoticed until it's almost too late. Regular mental health check-ins can be game-changers. Psychological assessments help catch early signs of conditions like depression, anxiety, and even cognitive decline. Being proactive about mental health involves more than just medicinal interventions; it can help tailor lifestyle choices that keep you in a balanced state of mind. When your mind is clear and focused, your ability to manage other aspects of health significantly improves.

Skin health is another area often overlooked but easily monitored. Regular self-exams and professional evaluations can catch skin cancer and other dermatological issues early. Be mindful of changes in moles or spots on your skin, and take action promptly. These simple habits can lead to early treatment and prevent more severe issues down the road.

Even dental check-ups play a pivotal role in your overall health. Oral health is deeply interconnected with heart health and other chronic conditions. Regular dental exams can intercept problems like gum disease, which has been linked to heart disease, diabetes, and even complications during pregnancy. It's a perfect example of how the various systems of our body are interconnected, and monitoring one aspect can have a ripple effect throughout your entire wellbeing.

Lab tests for thyroid function, vitamin levels, and hormonal balance can unmask underlying issues that manifest subtly but have long-term implications. Properly functioning thyroid levels, for example, regulate metabolism, energy levels, and even mood. Insufficient levels of essential vitamins and minerals can have far-reaching effects, from brittle bones to impaired cognitive function. Diagnosing and correcting these imbalances early can stave off more severe health issues down the road.

Combining these various strategies forms a robust preventive healthcare regime that supports longevity and enhances quality of life. Being habitual about getting these check-ups isn't about living in fear—it's about living smart. It's about taking responsibility for your own health and well-being, knowing that each early detection strategy is a step towards a healthier, more vibrant you.

We can't talk about early detection strategies without mentioning lifestyle choices. Smoking cessation programs, moderating alcohol intake, and maintaining a balanced diet can all help in early detection and prevention. These strategies not only contribute to immediate health benefits but also provide data points that help in early diagnosis. When a physician has a comprehensive view of your lifestyle habits, it allows them to offer more personalized and effective healthcare advice.

Building a proactive health routine involves setting reminders for these crucial tests and check-ups. Pencil them into your calendars like you would any other appointment. Many healthcare providers offer automated systems that can help remind you when it's time for your screenings. Embrace technology to help you stay on top of your health game. These reminders act as gentle nudges, urging you to take those pivotal steps towards early detection and consequently," healthier you

The essence of early detection lies in its ability to give you control over your health destiny. By incorporating these strategies into your regular healthcare routine, you're making a commitment to not just add years to your life but add life to your years. You're equipping yourself with the tools to catch potential issues in their infancy and empowering yourself with the ability to manage your health proactively.

Understanding that your health is an intricate tapestry woven from countless threads, each check-up, each test, each early detection strategy is like reinforcing those threads, ensuring the entire structure remains strong and resilient. This proactive stance is not only empowering but deeply inspiring. It's about respecting the body that carries you through life and giving it the attention and care it so richly deserves.

Chapter 10:
The Importance of Purpose and Passion

As we delve into the essence of living a longer, more vibrant life, it's essential to recognize the transformative power of purpose and passion. They're not just feel-good concepts; they're vital drivers of longevity. When you wake up each morning with a sense of purpose, your psychological and physiological systems align to support your well-being. Passion fuels resilience, providing the motivation to stay active, eat healthily, and foster meaningful connections. Research shows that individuals with a strong sense of purpose tend to have lower levels of stress and inflammation, both key factors in aging. Furthermore, passion isn't confined to grand pursuits; it can be found in everyday activities that bring joy and fulfillment. By cultivating a life rich in purpose and passion, you're not only adding years to your life but life to your years.

Finding Meaning in Life

Living a long, healthy life is about more than just eating well and exercising. At some point, most of us find ourselves questioning the deeper, more elusive aspects of our existence. Finding meaning in life is not merely a philosophical endeavor—it's a practical one that impacts our health and longevity.

Studies have shown that individuals who have a strong sense of purpose tend to outlive their counterparts who don't. But what does it mean to find meaning? It's as unique as our fingerprints. For some, it's about contributing to the community, for others, it might be raising a family, creating art, or advancing in their career. The key is that whatever stirs your soul must resonate deeply within you.

Purpose acts like a North Star, guiding you through life's challenges and joys. It can change and evolve, but having that direction is what fuels both your mind and body. When you wake up with a reason to get out of bed, it can drastically improve your mental health, thereby positively affecting your physical health. Simple as it sounds, feeling valuable and needed can keep ailments at bay.

Having a purpose doesn't mean avoiding difficulties—it means facing them with intent. When you know your 'why,' you become resilient. You see obstacles as part of your journey rather than insurmountable barriers. Cultivating this mindset is imperative for overall well-being.

Research suggests that people who have a sense of purpose are less likely to suffer from chronic illnesses, experience lower levels of stress, and even have healthier behaviors like regular exercise and balanced eating. It's a holistic cycle: your purpose drives healthier habits, which in turn, make it easier to fulfill your purpose.

One way to begin uncovering your purpose is to reflect on what genuinely excites you. Think about what activities or causes make you lose track of time. These moments, often aligned with your passions, can point you in the right direction. When you're deeply engaged in something that you care about, you're more likely to experience a state of flow—a psychological condition that's been linked to improved health and wellbeing.

Also, don't underestimate the power of small acts. Meaning doesn't always have to manifest in grand gestures. Sometimes, it's the little things, like helping a neighbor or volunteering at a local shelter, that add up to a significant impact. These actions create a ripple effect, not just in the community, but within you as well, enriching your own life as you enrich others'.

Communicating and connecting with others enriches our sense of purpose. Human beings are inherently social creatures and building meaningful relationships fuels a sense of belonging. These connections can be life-affirming and life-extending. They help us feel seen, heard, and valued, which is fundamental to our mental and physical health.

It's easy to assume that purpose and passion are solely individual quests. However, these can be social and communal endeavors that align with larger goals or shared experiences. This is especially relevant when facing life transitions, such as retirement or loss of a loved one, which may initially feel like big voids but can become opportunities to discover or recalibrate your purpose.

Everybody goes through phases where finding meaning seems elusive. During these times, it can be helpful to seek guidance. Whether through counseling, spirituality, or community engagement, external perspectives can illuminate paths that we might not see on our own. The journey to finding meaning is ongoing, rarely linear, and that's okay.

For those struggling to identify a sense of purpose, start simple and be kind to yourself. Practice gratitude, both for the journey and for the opportunities to discover what you're meant to do. As you begin to focus on what you have rather than what you lack, you'll find it easier to see the value in everyday moments.

Furthermore, integrating mindfulness and meditation practices can assist in this journey. Being present helps you connect with your true desires and aspirations. When we're mindful, we're more likely to notice what genuinely sparks joy and fulfillment in our lives.

Finding meaning in life and embracing your passions doesn't just extend your lifespan; it enriches the quality of your years. It creates a more vibrant, fulfilling existence that makes every day a gift rather than a grind. It's about thriving, not just surviving.

It's crucial to regularly reassess what gives you a sense of meaning. Life changes, and so do your circumstances, and with that, what you value may also shift. Responding to these changes with adaptability ensures that you stay aligned with your evolving sense of purpose.

It's worth noting that finding meaning doesn't require grandiose achievements. Small, intentional actions that align with your values can be profoundly meaningful. Whether it's walking in nature, mentoring a young professional, or simply being present for your loved ones, these acts accumulate and form a life rich in purpose. Remember, it's the heart and intention behind these actions that matter most.

In summary, finding meaning in life isn't just for philosophers and daydreamers—it's an essential component of a healthy, extended life. It offers a holistic approach to well-being that combines mental, physical, and emotional health. Lastly, understand that meaning is not static— it's a dynamic journey. Embrace it with open arms, and in doing so, you'll find that life becomes not just longer, but more profoundly enriching.

How Passion Contributes to Longevity

Passion is a powerhouse. When you're deeply passionate about something, you get into a state of flow where time seems to disappear, and you're fully immersed in what you love. This state not only elevates your mood but also has tangible health benefits that can add years to your life. The surge of positive emotions you feel when you're doing what you love lowers cortisol levels, which in turn decreases chronic stress – a known enemy of longevity.

Consider this: when you're passionate about something, be it gardening, painting, or even starting a small business, you generate a sense of purpose. Living with a sense of purpose has repeatedly been linked with better health outcomes. Studies show that individuals with a clear purpose in life are less likely to succumb to diseases like Alzheimer's and heart disease. The act of engaging in meaningful activities stimulates the brain, keeps it active, and even helps form new neural connections. Essentially, passion fuels your brain, keeping it young and dynamic.

Moreover, the physical manifestations of indulging in your passions shouldn't be overlooked. Think about the adrenaline rush, the dopamine spikes, and the general physical activity some passions require. Physical activity, even if not strenuous, promotes cardiovascular health, enhances flexibility, and helps maintain a healthy weight. All these factors collectively enhance your lifespan, creating a harmonious cycle between body and soul.

Passion also acts as a buffer against the wear and tear of daily life. Life throws curveballs, and while there's no way to avoid every hardship, the resilience built through passionate pursuits helps you bounce back more readily. People who are passionate about their activities often exhibit higher levels of resilience and optimism, two key factors in living a longer, more fulfilling life. This resilience can be incredibly beneficial during tough times, making it easier to navigate life's inevitable ups and downs.

Let's not forget the social aspect. Passion often brings people together, forming communities of like-minded individuals. Whether it's a book club, a dance class, or a local sports team, these communal settings foster social ties, which are crucial for mental and emotional well-being. Social connections have been shown to lower the risk of chronic conditions and mental illnesses. So, you're not just indulging in a hobby; you're also building a support network that bolsters your health and longevity.

Passion also keeps you curious, keeps you learning. Lifelong learning is another pillar of longevity. When you're passionate about something, you're likely to continuously seek out new information, new techniques, or even new challenges within that realm. This ongoing quest for knowledge keeps your brain adaptable, young, and vibrant, protecting against cognitive decline.

Furthermore, passion-driven individuals often report higher levels of life satisfaction and sense of accomplishment. This subtle yet powerful psychological state can deter the onset of anxiety and depression, which, if left unchecked, can negatively impact your overall health and longevity. The mind-body connection resonates profoundly here; a joyful mind often translates to a healthier body.

In fact, passion can even be seen as a preventive measure. Engaging deeply in activities you love acts as a natural form of self-care. Instead of seeing relaxation or personal time as indulgent, it becomes a necessary element of your well-being routine. By allowing yourself the freedom to pursue your interests, you're naturally allocating time for mental decompression and physical recovery, both of which are essential for long-term health.

In many ways, passion is like the core of an apple. It's central, yet often hidden, but it's vital for the fruit's growth and survival. While external factors like diet, exercise, and sleep play critical roles in longevity, the internal drive – your passion – can be equally important. It's the secret ingredient that gives you a zest for life, an energy that can be palpably felt and harnessed for longevity.

It's not about finding grandiose passions, either. Your passion doesn't have to be something that changes the world. It can be as simple as enjoying bird watching, writing poetry, or even collecting stamps. What matters is the personal joy and fulfillment that activity brings to you. When you're genuinely happy and engaged, hormones like endorphins and serotonin flood your system, creating a biochemical environment conducive to long life.

Moreover, passion is likely to keep you engaged with new techniques and technologies that can enhance and maintain your health. For instance, a passionate runner might be more inclined to learn about innovative footwear technology or breakthroughs in physical therapy that can aid in injury prevention and recovery. These small but significant steps contribute to continued physical well-being, reinforcing the powerful cycle of health and passion.

In conclusion, passion is a hidden wellspring of longevity. It's an intangible yet profound force that adds substance to your days, joy to your heart, and vitality to your body. When you find what makes you come alive, you're not just adding years to your life, but life to your years. So, dive into your passions, embrace them wholeheartedly, and watch as the vibrant dance of life prolongs your journey on this beautiful planet.

Chapter 11:
Real-Life Stories of Longevity

The world is teeming with inspiring individuals who've cracked the code to a long, healthy life, and their stories can teach us more than any clinical study. Imagine sitting across the table from a spry centenarian, sipping tea as they recount not just their years, but their intentional choices—simple yet profound decisions that led them to celebrate a century of vibrant living. One of these stories hails from the serene landscapes of Okinawa, where elders treasure community, purposeful activity, and a diet brimming with fresh, colorful produce. Another tale unfolds in the Mediterranean, where evenings are spent in the company of loved ones, savoring heart-healthy meals and laughter. These snapshots of longevity bring the concepts of healthy living out of the abstract and into the tangible, showing us that the path to a longer life is paved not just with nutritious food and consistent exercise, but also with connection, purpose, and joy. So, let these stories inspire you to embrace life with a renewed fervor, knowing that with each mindful choice, you're crafting your own legacy of longevity.

Interviews with Centenarians

Imagine sitting down with someone who has lived over a century. The stories they'd tell, the wisdom they'd share—it's like opening a time capsule filled with invaluable life lessons. Listening to their experiences isn't just enriching; it's also a potent reminder that the keys to longevity are often simple and accessible to us all.

Our first centenarian, Maria, lived to be 104. When asked about her secret to longevity, she laughed and said, "Simple pleasures and good company." Born in a small village in Italy, Maria moved to the United States in her twenties. Her days were filled with laughter, good food, and close family ties. "Every evening," she recounted, "we'd gather around the dinner table. It was noisy, but it was beautiful. We ate homemade bread, fresh vegetables from the garden, and fish from the local market. Nothing fancy, just fresh and real."

These moments, seemingly mundane, were foundational for Maria's long, vibrant life. It's easy to underestimate the power of such daily rituals, but these small, repeated actions build up over time. Her story tells us that good nutrition, a supportive environment, and emotional connections play essential roles in our longevity.

Another conversation brought us to John, a 101-year-old war veteran. John's life, filled with travel and adventure, was anything but ordinary. "I never stayed in one place too long," he told us, "I think that's what kept me young." John's perspective is an interesting one—it wasn't just the physical activity but the constant mental stimulation and adaptation that he believes kept him sharp. "You have to keep your mind engaged," he said, "whether it's learning a new language, picking up a hobby, or just meeting new people."

It's fascinating how each centenarian has unique principles yet underlying themes of community, diet, and mental stimulation are consistent. This was echoed by Evelyn, who celebrated her 102nd birthday by dancing with her great-grandchildren. Evelyn's focus was on the importance of maintaining her physical health through movement. "Every morning, I did a little dance, even if it was just in my living room," she laughed. Her eyes sparkled with a youthful energy that belied her years. "Movement is life," she insisted. Her grandchildren once set up a dance room for her, complete with soft floors and mirrors, and she'd spend hours there, moving to the rhythm of her life.

The role of stress—or rather, the management of stress—can't be ignored either. Centenarians like James, who lived until he was 108, swore by a stress-free lifestyle. "I let things go easily," he explained. "No point holding on to worries." James engaged in daily mindfulness practices long before they became mainstream. Techniques such as deep breathing, meditation, and even simple walks in nature featured heavily in his routine. These habits helped him maintain a serene and focused mind, a critical element of his longevity.

Nutrition cropped up again and again in our interviews but always in the context of balance and enjoyment. Take, for example, 100-year-old Sarah, who never denied herself a piece of her beloved dark chocolate. "It's about savoring life," she said. Sarah emphasized that joy from food is just as important as its nutritional value. "I never ate food I didn't like. Why would I?" This encapsulates the wisdom of enjoying indulgences in moderation rather than seeing them as forbidden.

One thing that stands out when talking to these centenarians is how they view food and exercise not as chores but as pleasures. They weren't counting calories or running marathons; they were eating vegetables from their gardens and taking long, leisurely walks. Their approach to health was integrated seamlessly into their lives—a model worth emulating.

Social connections were a cornerstone for each centenarian. Many of them lived in multi-generational homes where family was a constant presence. Emma, a 103-year-old grandmother, spoke of the regular gatherings hosted at her home. "Everyone came over at least once a week. There was always someone at the house, which made it lively and filled with laughter." Emma's life underscores the importance of social engagement and support networks, elements that numerous studies have linked to increased longevity.

No conversation on longevity would be complete without mentioning the role of purpose and passion. Felipe, who lived 102 years, spent each morning tending to his orchids. "They need love, care, and patience," he said, "just like people." Felipe's dedication to his flowers wasn't merely a hobby; it gave him a profound sense of purpose. Engaging in meaningful activities added zest to his life, not just in his twilight years, but throughout his entire lifespan.

The centenarians' wisdom is immensely valuable. They teach us that the most effective longevity strategies are often the most straightforward: eat well, stay active, manage stress, maintain social connections, and find meaning in your daily life. It's a tapestry of habits woven together to create a life that's not only long but deeply fulfilling.

Perhaps the most motivating insight from these interviews is how accessible these habits can be. There's a simplicity to the lives of these centenarians that stands in contrast to our often frenetic, modern lifestyle. Yet, it's precisely this simplicity that holds the key to their longevity. As you reflect on their stories, consider how you can integrate these timeless principles into your own life. Remember, the journey to a longer, healthier life starts with small, meaningful steps.

Equipped with these insights, you're better prepared to embrace a lifestyle that promotes longevity. Take inspiration from Maria, John, Evelyn, James, Sarah, Emma, and Felipe. Each of them exemplifies how the choices we make every day—and the attitude we bring to those choices—can profoundly impact our lifespan and, more importantly, our quality of life.

Lessons Learned from the Long-Lived

Stepping into the lives of those who've surpassed the century mark, you'll unearth an array of wisdom that transcends time and culture. Living longer isn't merely about adding more years to life, but about adding life to those years. Let's explore the gems of life lessons shared by the long-lived that can guide us on our journey to health and longevity in a way that's both inspirational and achievable.

One of the most profound lessons learned from centenarians is the importance of maintaining a positive outlook. Many people who've lived a hundred years or more often share stories about enduring adversity with a smile. It seems that seeing the glass as half full can indeed have tangible benefits on your lifespan. Optimism doesn't just change your day—it could change your years, adding more of them and filling them with joy.

The long-lived are masters of adaptability. Life throws curveballs at all of us, but those who've lived the longest have learned to roll with the punches. Flexibility in the face of change enhances mental resilience and reduces stress. This doesn't mean we should start expecting all changes to be easy, but rather embrace the mindset that we can navigate whatever life hands us. Just as a tree bends with the wind, so too can we learn to sway without breaking.

Another cornerstone of longevity is the cultivation of meaningful relationships. Numerous centenarians express that their connections with family, friends, and community have been pivotal. Building and nurturing these relationships not only provides emotional support but also offers practical help, reducing stress and increasing happiness. Social bonds act as buffers against the strains of life, and it's clear that we are wired to thrive through connection.

Purpose and passion go hand in hand with longevity. Many centenarians remain engaged in activities they love, even if those activities evolve over time. Whether it's gardening, painting, or volunteering, having a reason to wake up in the morning significantly contributes to both mental and physical health. Purpose is like the rudder of a ship, steering us through the waters of life and keeping us moving forward.

Diet, unsurprisingly, plays a crucial role. The long-lived often follow what we'd now identify as 'traditional diets'—rich in whole, unprocessed foods and low in sugar. Whether it's the Mediterranean diet abundant in olive oil and lean proteins or the plant-heavy diet of the Okinawans, these nutritional choices are a testament to the adage, "You are what you eat." Eating well fuels the body and nourishes the soul.

Exercise doesn't always mean hitting the gym; sometimes, it's as simple as staying active through daily routines. Centenarians tend to incorporate physical activity naturally into their lives rather than adhering to rigid workout schedules. Walking, gardening, and even light chores keep the body moving without feeling like a burden. The secret might just lie in consistency over intensity.

Let's not overlook the mental aspects of health. Many centenarians practice forms of mindfulness and meditation, whether through formal techniques or simply living in the moment. This cultivation of mental peace reduces stress and contributes to overall well-being. Sometimes it's okay to stop, breathe, and take in the world around you without rushing through it.

A noteworthy lesson involves the principle of moderation. Living long doesn't mean depriving oneself of pleasures but enjoying them in balance. A glass of wine here, a piece of chocolate there—small indulgences are part of a well-lived life when they're savored mindfully. This balanced approach extends to work and play, rest and activity, solitude and socializing. Balance, it seems, might be closer to a universal truth than we realized.

An element of spirituality or faith is often present among the long-lived. This isn't about adhering to a specific religion but rather having a set of beliefs or a framework that brings comfort and meaning. Spirituality provides mental and emotional fortitude, helping individuals cope with life's highs and lows. It's about having something greater than oneself to turn to, whether that's faith, nature, or philosophies.

Centenarians also demonstrate a certain zest for life that's infectious. They remain curious, open to learning, and passionate about exploring new things. Whether it's reading new books, learning a new craft, or simply staying updated with technology, this continuous engagement stimulates the brain and keeps the mind young.

Interestingly, many of the long-lived highlight the importance of routine. While some might view routines as restrictive, centenarians see them as a stabilizing force. Regular sleep patterns, meal times, and daily activities create a sense of normalcy and predictability that can fortify overall health. It's a reminder that structure doesn't necessarily stifle freedom; sometimes, it enhances it.

Lastly, let's talk gratitude. Many centenarians attribute their long lives to an attitude of gratefulness. Daily practices of acknowledging and appreciating the positives in life contribute to a content and fulfilling existence. Gratitude shifts focus from what's missing to what's there, creating an abundance mindset that can enhance well-being.

These lessons from the long-lived aren't magical formulas but practical guidelines that can be woven into our everyday lives. They invite us to slow down, cherish each day, and live fully with intention. These insights spark a journey rather than presenting an endpoint, encouraging us to continually adapt and grow.

Incorporating these timeless truths into your life doesn't require a complete overhaul. Start small: engage in activities that make you happy, surround yourself with a supportive community, and maintain a balanced diet. Pay attention to your mental health, keep active in ways you enjoy, and cultivate an attitude of gratitude. After all, it's often the simplest shifts that lead to the most profound changes in our health and longevity.

Through the eyes of those who've walked long before us, life reveals itself not as a race to the end but as a rich tapestry of experiences and connections. Embrace the lessons imparted by our centenarians, and you may find yourself not only living longer but living better.

Chapter 12:
Actionable Tips for
Everyday Living

Imagine infusing your everyday life with simple yet powerful habits that can dramatically enhance your health and longevity. Start your morning with a routine that invigorates both body and mind - maybe it's a few minutes of meditation followed by a nutritious breakfast. Small changes, like staying hydrated throughout the day and snatching moments for mindfulness, anchor your wellbeing in the present. As evening comes, embrace a wind-down period to signal your body it's time to rest; think tranquil activities like reading or gentle stretching. It's also vital to regularly evaluate and set tangible health goals to keep your journey towards longevity on track. These everyday choices are your toolkit for a vibrant, long life - so make them count, and you'll feel the difference with every step.

Daily Habits for a Healthier Life

Transforming your everyday routines can be a game-changer for your health and longevity. Start small with habits like drinking a glass of water first thing in the morning and gradually incorporating more intentional practices into your day. Mix regular physical activity with moments of mindfulness, like taking deep breaths while brewing your morning coffee or practicing gratitude while brushing your teeth. Balance your diet with nutrient-dense foods and make an effort to minimize screen time, especially before bed. A consistent sleep schedule, coupled with a mindful evening routine, can work wonders for your overall well-being. Take moments throughout the day to stand, stretch, and move your body—simple actions that add up over time. Building these daily habits isn't just about adding years to your life but enriching the quality of those years. Let each day be a step towards a more vibrant and fulfilled you.

Morning Routines are the heartbeat of our day; they set the rhythm and tempo for the hours to come. When you begin your morning with intention, you pave the way for a day filled with vitality and purpose. If you've ever wondered about the secrets to a long, healthy life, it might surprise you that much of it starts as the sun begins to rise.

Imagine waking up gently, with the first rays of sunlight filtering through your curtains. This simple act ties back to our biological rhythms. Our bodies are designed to wake up with the sun, thanks to our circadian rhythms. Exposure to natural light early in the day can improve mood, increase alertness, and even help regulate sleep patterns. It's not just about rolling out of bed; it's about connecting with the world as it awakens.

Starting your day with hydration is crucial. After a night of fasting, your body craves water. Drinking a glass of water in the morning kickstarts your metabolism, flushes out toxins, and hydrates your cells. Some people add a squeeze of lemon for an extra boost of Vitamin C and a slight detoxifying effect. It's a small, but powerful habit that nourishes every cell in your body.

Another cornerstone of a healthy morning routine is movement. This doesn't mean you need an elaborate workout first thing, though. Gentle stretching, a short yoga session, or even a quick walk can activate your muscles, improve circulation, and get your body ready for the day. Physical activity in the morning can also boost endorphins, those feel-good hormones that set a positive tone for the entire day.

Making movement part of your morning establishes a precedent: today, your health is a priority.

Nutrition in the morning cannot be overlooked. A balanced breakfast serves as the foundation for your daily fuel. Incorporate protein, healthy fats, and fiber to keep your energy levels stable. Think avocado toast, smoothie bowls with nuts and seeds, or a simple vegetable omelet. The goal is to avoid sugar crashes that can occur with high-carb breakfasts. Instead, nourish your body with wholesome foods that support sustained energy and focus.

Tuning into your mental health as part of your morning routine is equally important. Practice mindfulness or meditation to center yourself. Even five minutes of being present can make a world of difference. These practices reduce stress, enhance mental clarity, and improve emotional well-being. It's wonderful to start the day with a clear mind, ready to handle whatever comes your way.

A morning routine should also include some form of mental stimulation. Read a book, solve a puzzle, or engage in another activity that challenges your brain. Mental flexibility and cognitive health are key elements of longevity. By nurturing your brain early in the day, you're preparing it for maximum performance and resilience throughout life's challenges.

Consider journaling as a powerful morning practice. Writing down your thoughts, goals, and gratitude can orient your mindset towards positivity and productivity. Reflecting on what you're thankful for has been shown to boost mood and overall life satisfaction, creating a ripple effect that lasts all day. It's a simple practice, but its benefits are profound.

Connecting with loved ones can also be a wonderful way to start the day. A quick chat with a family member or even a heartfelt message to a friend can uplift your spirits. Human connections add a layer of emotional richness and support that is invaluable for long-term health and happiness.

Your environment plays a significant role in your morning routine, too. Creating a serene, clutter-free space can make your morning feel less chaotic and more purposeful. Small touches like a clean kitchen counter for breakfast prep or a dedicated corner for meditation can enhance your morning routine. Aesthetics matter — they influence your mood and stress levels more than you might realize.

Incorporating learning into your morning can also be transformational. Listen to a podcast, watch an educational video, or read a chapter from a book that interests you. Learning something new each day keeps your brain young and agile. It's an investment in your intellectual growth that pays dividends as you age.

If your mornings tend to be rushed, focus on creating a routine that's realistic and achievable. Set aside 30 minutes for these intentional activities. This might mean waking up a bit earlier, but it's a small sacrifice for the immense benefits it brings. Preparation the night before can also make your morning smoother. Lay out your clothes, prep breakfast ingredients, or write down your to-do list. These small steps can make your mornings feel less encumbered and more controlled.

Guard your morning time jealously. It's your sacred space to establish the tone for a day of wellness and productivity. Avoid diving into emails or social media right away. These distractions can derail your intentions and pull you into reactive mode. Instead, focus on activities that ground you and set a positive trajectory for your day.

The benefits of a well-crafted morning routine cannot be overstated. It's not just about the physical actions; it's about cultivating a mindset where health and longevity are non-negotiable priorities. Each morning is a new opportunity to make choices that support a long, vibrant life. Embrace it.

As we delve deeper into these daily habits, you'll see that a disciplined morning routine is often where health transformations begin. It's the first step, the foundation upon which the rest of the day is built. When you commit to a mindful morning, you are setting the stage for a life well-lived, rich in health, joy, and purpose.

Evening Wind-Downs are an integral part of a holistic approach to optimizing your health and longevity. As the day draws to a close, it's essential to set the stage for restful sleep and recharge your mind and body for the day ahead. Evening routines are about more than just unwinding; they're a bridge between the day's takings and a good night's sleep, setting you up for a restful night and an energized morning.

One of the simplest yet most overlooked methods to wind down is by dimming the lights. As natural sunlight fades into twilight, artificial lighting can trick your brain into thinking it's still daytime. By dimming the lights at home, you're signaling your body to produce melatonin, the hormone responsible for regulating sleep. This small adjustment acts as a natural cue to prepare for rest, making your transition to sleep much smoother.

Another key component is to disconnect from electronic devices. Our gadgets emit blue light, which can interfere with melatonin production and disturb your circadian rhythm. Scrolling through your phone or watching TV right before bed can be particularly disruptive. Try to limit your screen time at least an hour before you intend to sleep. Instead, opt for calming activities such as reading a book, journaling your thoughts, or engaging in a creative hobby.

Engaging in a relaxing activity can greatly enhance your evening wind-down. Consider adopting a short evening meditation or gentle yoga practice. Both of these activities help relax the mind and body, reducing stress levels and preparing your body for sleep. Even just a few minutes of mindful breathing can make a profound difference in your overall sense of well-being.

Complement your winding-down activities with a warm drink, preferably non-caffeinated. Herbal teas like chamomile, peppermint, or lavender are excellent choices. Sipping on a warm, soothing beverage can help relax your muscles and mind, creating the perfect ambiance for sleep.

Establishing a nightly skincare routine can also signal to your body that it's time to wind down. Cleansing your face, applying a moisturizer, and possibly a nighttime serum not only benefits your skin but also offers a few quiet moments to reflect on your day. This self-care ritual can become a cherished part of your evening, promoting both relaxation and self-love.

Maintaining a consistent bedtime is crucial. The human body thrives on routine, and going to bed at the same time each night helps regulate your internal clock. Ensure that your bedtime allows you at least seven to eight hours of sleep, which is optimal for most adults. Consistency fosters a stronger circadian rhythm, making it easier to fall asleep and wake up naturally.

Let's not forget the importance of your bedroom environment. Keep your sleeping space cool, quiet, and dark to promote restful sleep. Consider investing in heavy curtains or a sleep mask to block out light, and use earplugs or a white noise machine if noise is an issue. Your bedroom should be a sanctuary for rest and relaxation, free from distractions and clutter.

One of the most potent ways to wind down is through ritual. Create a series of small, repetitive actions that cue your mind and body that it's time to sleep. This could be as simple as laying out your clothes for the next day, fluffing your pillows, or turning down the bedcovers. These small actions, when done consistently, can build a powerful association with sleep.

If you struggle with falling asleep, guided visualization can be an effective tool. Picture a serene landscape or a comforting scenario in your mind. This mental escape helps divert your focus from daily worries and anxieties, transitioning you into a more peaceful state conducive to sleep. Likewise, if persistent thoughts keep you awake, jot them down on a notepad beside your bed. Offloading these thoughts can provide mental relief and pave the way for a quieter mind.

Physical relaxation techniques such as progressive muscle relaxation can be incredibly beneficial. Starting from your toes and working your way up to your head, tense and then release each muscle group. This practice can alleviate physical tension and promote a deeper sense of relaxation, making it easier to drift off to sleep.

Lifestyle adjustments can also play an important role. Avoid heavy meals and alcohol close to bedtime, as they can disrupt your sleep cycle. If you're hungry before bed, opt for a light snack, such as a banana or a handful of almonds, both of which contain sleep-supportive nutrients like magnesium and tryptophan.

Aromatherapy can provide an added layer of comfort. Essential oils such as lavender, chamomile, and cedarwood are known for their calming properties. You can use a diffuser to disperse these scents throughout your room or apply a few drops to your pillow. The soothing aromas can help quiet your mind and prepare your senses for sleep.

Finally, cultivating appreciation before bed can have a profound impact on your mental state. Take a moment to reflect on what you're grateful for, to acknowledge even the smallest wins of the day, or to simply appreciate the calmness of the night. Gratitude practices not only improve your overall mood but also create a positive mental environment for sleep.

In the quest for longevity and optimal health, **Evening Wind-Downs** are an invaluable part of the equation. By blending simple, mindful practices into your nightly routine, you can transform your evenings from a chaotic end to a harmonious conclusion, fostering better sleep and promoting overall well-being. These habits may seem small, but their cumulative effect can significantly enhance your quality of life.

Goal Setting for Longevity

Goal setting can often feel like that one persistent item on your to-do list that never quite gets checked off. But when it comes to longevity, setting the right goals is not just a nice-to-have—it's essential. If we're serious about living longer, healthier lives, then we need to take goal setting seriously too.

First things first: let's define what we mean by "goal setting for longevity." At its core, it's about making deliberate, actionable plans— big and small—that can help us improve our lifespan and overall quality of life. We're talking about establishing daily routines, lifestyle changes, and milestones that collectively contribute towards a healthier, longer life.

Maybe you've heard the saying, "What gets measured gets managed." It's spot-on when it comes to achieving long-term health objectives. Identifying specific, measurable goals is crucial. For instance, instead of vaguely aiming to "exercise more," commit to something concrete. Say, "I will walk 10,000 steps a day," or "I'll do strength training three times a week." This specificity helps track progress and make adjustments as needed.

So, why do goals matter so much? They act as north stars, guiding your actions day in and day out. When we lay out clear, attainable goals, we build momentum, which solidifies habits over time. And trust, these small, daily victories create a domino effect, leading to bigger wins in the long run.

One often overlooked aspect of goal setting is breaking down long-term goals into manageable chunks. Think of it as building a ladder with each rung representing a small, achievable step. For longevity, these could be yearly check-ups, quarterly health reviews, or even monthly new habits. By stacking up these smaller goals, you can climb closer to your ultimate objective of a longer, healthier life.

It's also worth noting the importance of flexibility in your goal-setting journey. Life is unpredictable. We get busy, plans change, or maybe an unexpected event throws us off course. The key is not to abandon your goals, but to adapt them as needed. Maybe you missed your daily exercise—don't stress. Instead, focus on eating a balanced meal or getting extra sleep. Your longevity goals should serve as guides, not rigid mandates.

Next, let's talk about the impact of a supportive environment. We are social creatures, and our circles significantly influence us. Share your goals with family and friends. Encourage them to join you. Having a support network can motivate you to stay on track and even make the journey more enjoyable. Surrounding yourself with people who share similar aspirations can transform a solo endeavor into a communal experience.

Another pillar in goal setting for longevity is continual reassessment. Did you know that even elite athletes and top performers regularly review and adjust their goals? You should too. Take time to evaluate what's working and what's not. Maybe you've been tracking your water intake religiously but realized sleep is a bigger challenge. Adjust your focus based on these insights.

The benefits of setting goals for longevity extend beyond physical health. Mental and emotional well-being are crucial components of a long, fulfilling life. Goals related to stress management, mindfulness, and emotional health are just as critical. Simple practices like setting aside time for meditation, engaging in hobbies you love, or even scheduling regular breaks during work can make a huge difference.

Incorporating variety into your goals can combat stagnation and keep things interesting. Try new exercises, experiment with different diets, or explore new hobbies. This not only keeps you engaged but also gives you a broader toolkit for longevity. Plus, it makes the process of achieving your goals more enjoyable and less of a chore.

And finally, celebrate your successes, no matter how small. Every step forward is a win. Did you hit your water intake goal for a week? Awesome. Walked every day this month? Fantastic. These micro-celebrations reinforce your dedication and help maintain your enthusiasm.

To wrap it all up, think of goal setting for longevity as a roadmap to a better, longer life. It's about taking incremental, purposeful steps that collectively bring you closer to your ultimate destination. By setting clear, actionable, and flexible goals, you build a foundation that supports not just your lifespan, but your healthspan—the quality of those extra years.

Setting goals is only the beginning. The real power lies in the execution, the daily actions, and the willingness to adapt and grow. It's a journey, after all, but one that promises rich rewards: more vibrant, healthier, and meaningful years ahead.

Conclusion

As we come to the end of this journey, it's time to reflect on the powerful tools and insights we've gathered to optimize our health and extend our lifespan. We've ventured through the intricate pathways of longevity, uncovering scientific truths and timeless wisdom. Now, it's up to each of us to apply these principles in our daily lives.

The science of longevity has given us invaluable understanding of how our bodies age and the biomarkers that influence this process. This foundational knowledge is crucial because it empowers us to make informed choices about our health. It's not just about adding years to our life, but life to our years. When we comprehend the mechanics of aging, we control our destiny to some extent.

Moreover, the role of nutrition in promoting a long and healthy life cannot be overstated. The shift towards whole foods, rich in antioxidants and anti-inflammatory nutrients, serves as a cornerstone for our well-being. Superfoods and fasting strategies further enhance our metabolic health, providing the energy and resilience we need to thrive. Our food choices don't merely sustain us; they can transform us. To integrate these dietary habits into our everyday routine is to choose a path of vitality and longevity.

Exercise and physical activity, royal regimens of any longevity plan, offer unmatched benefits. Whether through cardiovascular exercises, strength training, or maintaining flexibility and balance, the landscape of movement is vast and varied. Regular physical activity fortifies our bodies and sharpens our minds, cultivating a robustness that reverberates through every aspect of our existence. Remember, moving is not just about burning calories; it's about celebrating life.

Yet, we must also tend to our mental gardens. Health isn't merely a physical endeavor. Stress management, quality sleep, and practices such as mindfulness and meditation are pillars that uphold our mental fortitude. Stress may be an unavoidable part of life, but managing it effectively can turn potential roadblocks into stepping stones. Sleep, often undervalued, is a critical element of rejuvenation. It's where our bodies and minds reset, preparing us to face a new day with vigor.

Human connection adds another layer to our wellbeing. Building a supportive network and addressing the impacts of loneliness can have profound effects on our health. We are inherently social creatures, and nurturing our relationships can significantly enhance our quality of life. The warmth of a close-knit community, the shared laughter and empathy, these are not just pleasant; they are vital for our longevity.

Environmental factors also play a significant role in our health. Creating a toxin-free home environment and minimizing exposure to harmful substances are simple yet effective ways to promote well-being. Small adjustments in our immediate surroundings can lead to substantial health benefits.

The marriage of ancient wisdom and modern science offers a holistic approach to health. Traditional medicine practices, when integrated with contemporary scientific knowledge, provide comprehensive strategies for well-being. This synthesis allows us to benefit from the best of both worlds, using ancient principles to enhance modern lifestyles.

Moreover, the advent of personalized medicine has revolutionized how we approach our health. Genetic testing and tailored health protocols afford us the opportunity to create highly individualized strategies. By understanding our unique genetic makeup, we can adopt preventative measures that are specifically suited to our needs, thereby optimizing our health landscape on a deeply personal level.

Preventative healthcare underlines this proactive approach. Regular check-ups and early detection strategies allow us to catch potential health issues before they become serious. The adage "an ounce of prevention is worth a pound of cure" rings particularly true. Proactive management can decrease the likelihood of chronic diseases and improve our quality of life significantly.

And let's not forget the driving forces of purpose and passion. Finding meaning in life and pursuing passions are not mere luxuries; they are health necessities. They give us a reason to wake up each morning with zest, fostering a psychological environment where both mind and body flourish. Purpose and passion are profound contributors to longevity, fueling our journey with enthusiasm and fulfillment.

Real-life stories of centenarians provide us with lived testimonials that these principles aren't just theories but tangible realities. These individuals exemplify the benefits of a longevity-focused lifestyle, offering a living blueprint of what's possible. Their experiences teach us that a combination of good habits, strong relationships, and a joyful spirit can lead to a long, fulfilling life.

The actionable tips we've discussed throughout this book are not meant to be overwhelming mandates but rather gentle suggestions to incorporate into your routine. Morning routines that set a positive tone for the day, evening wind-downs that promote restful sleep, and goal setting that keeps you motivated and aligned with your health aspirations.

And so, we stand at the cusp of transformation. The knowledge and tools you've acquired are the seeds. It's now up to you to plant these seeds, nurture them, and watch them grow. Your journey towards longevity is not a rigid path but a dynamic adventure, filled with opportunities for growth, learning, and joy.

Empower yourself with this wisdom. Let each choice be a testament to your commitment to living a longer, healthier, and more fulfilling life. The journey of a thousand miles begins with a single step. So, take that step today. Dive into the fullness of life with a heart full of curiosity and a spirit eager for growth. Live not just long, but well.

Your life—full of visions, dreams, and boundless potential—is the greatest journey of all. Embrace it, cherish it, and make every moment count.

Appendix A:
Appendix

Welcome to the appendix, a curated collection of additional resources designed to supplement your journey toward optimal health and longevity. This section functions as a bridge, connecting you with further reading materials, cutting-edge research, and useful tools that can elevate your understanding and implementation of the concepts discussed throughout the book. Your proactive steps toward a healthier, longer life soar higher when bolstered by the right resources.

Recommended Resources

In the following list, you'll find books, articles, websites, and tools that have been personally vetted for their quality and relevance. Each resource has been selected to provide deeper insights, practical advice, or innovative approaches to health and longevity.

Books

"The Blue Zones: Lessons for Living Longer from the People Who've Lived the Longest" by Dan Buettner - An illuminating look into regions of the world where people live measurably longer lives.

"Lifespan: Why We Age—and Why We Don't Have To" by Dr. David Sinclair - A groundbreaking exploration of the science and potential of anti-aging.

"How Not to Die: Discover the Foods Scientifically Proven to Prevent and Reverse Disease" by Dr. Michael Greger - A vital handbook outlining the importance of nutrition and lifestyle changes.

Websites

WebMD - www.webmd.com - Comprehensive information on various health topics based on medical expertise.

National Institute on Aging - www.nia.nih.gov - Research and practical advice directly from experts.

Mayo Clinic - www.mayoclinic.org - Authoritative insights into symptoms, causes, and treatments of medical conditions.

Tools and Apps

MyFitnessPal - A versatile app that helps you track your diet and exercise habits.

Headspace - A mindfulness app offering guided meditations and wellness tips to improve mental health.

Sleep Cycle - An intelligent alarm clock that analyzes your sleep patterns and wakes you up in the lightest sleep phase for optimal rest.

Never underestimate the power of continued learning. The more informed you are, the more empowered you'll feel to make decisions that positively impact your health and well-being. These additional resources are here to help you delve deeper and embrace a lifestyle that aligns with your aspirations for longevity and vitality.

Remember, the journey toward a healthier, longer life is an exciting one. With the foundation laid out in this book and the supplementary resources provided herein, you're well-equipped to embark on this transformative path.

Final Thoughts

Every step you take, no matter how small, contributes to a healthier, more vibrant future. Use these resources as stepping stones, guiding and supporting you along the way. Let's make the most of this beautiful journey together, embracing the knowledge, wisdom, and tools available to us.

Here's to a life filled with health, happiness, and longevity!

Recommended Resources

In our quest for optimal health and longevity, the right resources can make all the difference. Whether you're just starting on your health journey or looking to deepen your existing knowledge, there are numerous books, websites, apps, and community groups that can provide invaluable support and information. Below, I've assembled an assortment of resources that cover a wide array of topics discussed throughout this book. These resources are carefully curated to help you unlock the secrets to a longer, healthier life.

First, let's dive into the world of books. When it comes to literature on health, nutrition, and longevity, countless titles offer insightful perspectives and practical advice. Consider starting with books by renowned experts in the field. Many of these authors blend scientific research with actionable steps you can incorporate into your daily life. Additionally, autobiographies and memoirs from individuals who have successfully implemented longevity principles can offer both inspiration and practical tips. Your local library or bookstore is a treasure trove of such wisdom.

For those more inclined to digital media, various websites and online platforms serve as excellent sources of information. Websites dedicated to health and wellness, like WebMD and Mayo Clinic, offer evidence-based articles and updates on the latest research. Additionally, some platforms specialize in specific areas like nutrition, exercise, or mental health. Subscribing to their newsletters can keep you abreast of new findings and emerging trends. Online forums and communities can also provide support and motivation from like-minded individuals on similar health journeys.

Next up are mobile apps, which can be particularly useful for tracking your progress and staying organized. There are numerous apps designed to monitor your diet, exercise routines, sleep patterns, and even stress levels. Apps like MyFitnessPal, Headspace, and Sleep Cycle provide a wealth of data right at your fingertips, empowering you to make informed decisions about your health. Many of these apps also offer personalized recommendations based on your inputs, helping you tailor your activities to meet your specific needs.

Social media channels can also be surprisingly effective tools for health and longevity. Following experts in the field on platforms like Instagram, Twitter, and LinkedIn can provide daily doses of inspiration and valuable tips. These platforms often host live Q&A sessions, webinars, and workshops that allow you to engage directly with experts. Just be cautious and ensure the information comes from credible sources; not every influencer is thoroughly vetted or qualified to give health advice.

Documentaries and podcasts are other fantastic resources, especially for those who prefer consuming information in an audio-visual format. Platforms like Netflix, Amazon Prime, and YouTube host numerous documentaries that explore various aspects of health, longevity, and wellness. Meanwhile, podcasts can be a convenient way to learn while you're on the go—whether you're commuting, exercising, or doing household chores. Shows like "The Joe Rogan Experience," "The Tim Ferriss Show," and "The Doctor's Farmacy" often feature renowned guests who delve into their areas of expertise.

Community and Support Groups: One often-overlooked resource is the power of community. Support groups, whether virtual or in-person, can provide emotional and moral backing that significantly impacts your motivation and adherence to healthy behaviors. Organizations like Meetup and local fitness clubs often sponsor health-focused events and group activities. Participating in these can foster a sense of belonging and keep you accountable to your goals.

For those interested in delving deeper into scientific literature, academic journals are invaluable resources. Journals such as "The New England Journal of Medicine," "The Lancet," and "Journal of the American Medical Association (JAMA)" are highly respected and offer the latest findings in health research. While these articles are often technical, they provide a rigorous examination of studies and trials that can be enlightening for those interested in the detailed science behind longevity.

Workshops and Conferences: Attending workshops, seminars, and conferences can also be extremely beneficial. These events often feature a range of speakers who are experts in their fields, offering an opportunity to learn from the best. Additionally, they provide a platform for networking with other health-conscious individuals. Many conferences are now available online, making them accessible no matter where you are.

Let's not forget the value of one-on-one guidance from professionals. From nutritionists and dietitians to personal trainers and mental health counselors, working directly with an expert can provide personalized advice tailored to your unique needs. Don't hesitate to invest in professional guidance if it's within your means; individualized advice can sometimes make all the difference in successfully implementing lifestyle changes.

Local community resources should not be overlooked. Community centers often offer classes and workshops on various aspects of health and wellness. Additionally, your local library can be a resource hub, offering books, DVDs, and sometimes even free health classes or talks. Checking community bulletin boards can reveal hidden gems close to home.

For those interested in traditional and alternative medicine, resources specializing in holistic approaches can be highly beneficial. Books and websites dedicated to Ayurveda, Traditional Chinese Medicine (TCM), and other ancient practices often offer a different perspective on health and wellbeing. Integrating this knowledge with modern medical advice can provide a balanced approach to longevity.

Healthcare System Resources: Your healthcare provider can also be an excellent resource. Regular check-ups allow you to monitor your health metrics and get professional advice based on your specific conditions. Many health insurance providers offer wellness programs that can include gym membership discounts, weight loss programs, and smoking cessation programs, so it's always worth exploring what's available to you.

Finally, always stay curious and open-minded. The field of health and longevity is constantly evolving, with new research and methodologies emerging regularly. Continued learning and adaptation can ensure you're always on the cutting edge of what's possible in the quest for a longer, healthier life. Remember that your journey to optimal health and longevity is unique to you, and the best resources are those that resonate most with your personal goals and lifestyle.

Choosing the right combination of resources can empower you to take proactive steps toward a healthier, longer life. From books and websites to apps and support groups, there's a wealth of information available to guide you on this journey. Explore these resources, find what works best for you, and let your commitment to health and longevity be ever-increasing.

Glossary of Terms

Welcome to our "Glossary of Terms"! This is your go-to list to understand the key concepts, jargon, and important phrases that we cover in this book.

Antioxidants - Compounds found in food that can prevent or delay some types of cell damage. They're often found in fruits and vegetables.

Biomarkers - Biological measures that can indicate a health condition or disease presence. For longevity, these can include blood pressure, cholesterol levels, and gene markers.

Cardiovascular Health - The health of the heart and blood vessels, crucial for overall longevity and physical well-being.

Dietary Fasting - Periods when you abstain from eating, which can have various health benefits such as improving metabolic functions and extending lifespan.

Holistic Approaches - Systems of health care that consider the whole person (body, mind, spirit) rather than just focusing on individual symptoms or illnesses.

Inflammation - The body's response to injury or infection, often manifesting as redness, swelling, or pain. Chronic inflammation can contribute to many diseases.

Longevity - The length of time that an individual lives. Strategies to promote longevity focus on extending both lifespan and healthspan.

Mindfulness - The practice of being present and fully engaged with whatever we're doing at the moment, free from distraction or judgment, and aware of our thoughts and feelings.

Nutrition - The process of providing or obtaining the food necessary for health and growth. In this context, it focuses on whole foods and nutrient-dense options to promote a long life.

Personalized Medicine - Medical practices that use genetic, environmental, and lifestyle factors to tailor health care to individual patients.

Superfoods - Nutrient-rich foods that are particularly beneficial for health and well-being. Examples include blueberries, kale, and salmon.

Traditional Medicine - Healing practices and therapies that have been passed down through generations, often rooted in cultural traditions.

Feel free to refer back to this glossary whenever you need a quick refresher on the terms we're discussing. Understanding these concepts will empower you to take control of your health and longevity journey!

www.ingramcontent.com/pod-product-compliance
Lightning Source LLC
Chambersburg PA
CBHW051429280526
45785CB00003B/1214